Trapped

The Nigel Logan Action Series #8

Kirk S. Jockell

The Free Mullet Press, LLC

ISBN: 978-1-963656-10-7 (paperback version)

Book Design by The Free Mullet Press, LLC

Cover Photo by Cover2Book.com

Author Photo by Debbie Hooper Photography

For Jan Lee

Since the earliest days of my writing journey, she has selflessly offered her eye, criticism, and wisdom to my work. Her contributions have helped shape and hone my skills as an author. Thank you, Jan.

Chapter One

A brave but nervous charter captain eased *Mare Stella*, his forty-one-foot fishing boat, through the channel and into Bahia de Cienfuegos, acting as if everything was normal. As did his passengers. Ignorance is bliss and proved positive as a port patrol boat moved alongside. Two of the passengers opened the big cooler, and both lifted a nice yellowfin tuna to show off as they grinned from ear to ear. Ernesto, the skipper, swallowed hard as he feigned a friendly smile, gave a thumbs up, and waved. The patrol boat crew waved back and continued, as Ernesto's breathing returned.

As he eased along, he looked up at the hillside. Castillo de Jagua stood watch over him and his vessel, the historic eighteenth-century fortress with its big cannons. It once protected the waters and the city of Cienfuegos. In the old days, sentries would scrutinize his every move. Now it is simply a museum and a tourist attraction. He turned back for a casual glance at the patrol boat. The waters are now protected by a much swifter and less forgiving force.

The passengers from Canada thought nothing of it when another boat approached and asked Ernesto to transport back to the marina a crew member who wasn't feeling well. Already knowing how the kind and friendly Canadians would react, he held up a finger and explained to his passengers the situation and asked their permission. "Of course," said the leader of the party that had booked the trip. "By all means, poor man."

They made the transfer; first a duffel bag, then his legs swung over the gunnel, and he dropped to the deck. He kept his head down and went below, but not before looking at Ernesto, nodding, and saying, "Gracias, el Capitan."

Ernesto nodded back, and the stranger disappeared.

Ernesto backed into his slip at Marlin Marina. Wives waited on the dock and waved enthusiastically to greet their husbands, who again lifted their catch to show how they had conquered the sea.

After Ernesto carried the catch to the cleaning station, he made quite the presentation of swiftly and most efficiently cleaning the fish. He held everyone's undivided attention, but from the corner of his eye, he caught his additional cargo slip off the boat and onto the dock. The man wore a big floppy hat as he slung the duffel over his shoulder and walked away, never looking back. Ernesto was happy about that and went back to his work. With another quick look, he saw the man turn a corner. *Buena suerte, señor.*

The man walked along the road with confidence, neither rushing nor taking his time. While he had never stayed there, he was all too familiar with the hostel he had been instructed to visit. The key was making the short four-block trip without being recognized.

As he turned up the walkway toward the front steps, a man came rushing out, took the duffle, and swiftly escorted the guest to the front door. He held it open as the man in the hat entered, then before following his guest, he gave a cursory glance around to make sure nobody had followed. Satisfied, he ducked inside and closed the door.

The two men looked at each other, and the owner of the hostel spoke first. "Bienvenido, Dr. Cabrera. I am..."

The doctor raised his hand. "No names, señor. I don't want to know. It is best that way."

The other man nodded in agreement as a handsome woman approached. The doctor gave a slight bow to express his appreciation. "Gracias, to you both."

"It is our pleasure," said the man. "She will now show you to your room. Please get comfortable. I know you must be tired."

"Si, indeed."

The doctor followed the woman until she opened a door and gestured for him to enter. She followed.

"Are you hungry, sir?"

"I am, but I am more tired than any hunger pang. I will rest now and take something later, if it pleases the señora?"

She nodded with a smile and said, "That will be fine." Then she shut the door.

He sat on the edge of the bed and looked around the room. He kicked his shoes off and swung his legs around so he could lie back. Before sleep consumed him, he whispered a prayer of gratitude. "Thank you, Lord. So far, so good."

The doctor couldn't decide what he enjoyed more, the meal of vaca frita, moros y cristianos, and sweet plantains, or his freshly bathed body and clean clothes. If he had to pick, being clean would probably top the list. And that says a lot, because the home-cooked food was exceptional.

The dangerous and covert trip from Barquisimeto, Venezuela, had been slow and tiring, and he wished he could feel happy to be back in his homeland. But that wasn't the case. As much as he once loved his country, despite all its corruption and problems, it had finally betrayed him and his family. His family was all he had left, and he wanted nothing more than to put it all back together again. With luck, timely action, and the grace and mercy of his Lord, they would all be together soon.

The man of the hostel saw a single flash of headlamps, a pause, and two more. He got up and peeked out the window. "The taxi is here." Turning around, he said, "It is time, doctor."

Dr. Cabrera stood and bowed toward his hosts. "And the adventure continues. Thank you for everything."

The men shook hands. Then the señora approached, got on her toes, and kissed the doctor on the cheek. Bouncing back on her heels, she said, "Por suerte. For luck."

"Gracias, señora."

The doctor grabbed his duffle and approached the door. Pulling the curtain, he looked and examined the 1958 Chevy Bel Air waiting beneath a streetlight. It was white and turquoise, just as he expected. Any other color would be disastrous, indicating trouble and the need to slip out the back, run, and make the best of it. Instead, he opened the door and slipped out. He opened the passenger side door, tossed the duffle in the backseat, and got in. The doctor looked at the driver who was smiling back. "Carlos," said the doctor, "it is so good to see you."

They leaned toward each other and exchanged a tight hug. Carlos patted the doctor on the back and said, "And the same for me, Alejandro. Hopefully, this will all be over soon."

They broke their embrace, and the doctor said, "Come on. Let's go."

They rode quietly through town on Paseo del Prado, the road that would lead them to Autopista 112 and further on to Palmira. Alejandro peered through the passenger window. "I wish I could see it in the daylight," he said, referring to his town. "Is it still as beautiful as I remember it?"

"You and Benita have been gone, what, four years?"

"It seems like forever."

"Well, a city over two hundred years old can only change so much. It is still the Pearl of the South."

"The Paris of Cuba," said Alejandro.

"Have you heard from Benita?"

Alejandro got quiet for a spell and Carlos didn't press.

"No. I have not. All I know is she works at a clinic in Belize, on the Placencia Peninsula."

"Does she know what you are doing?"

Alejandro turned to look at his friend. "No." Then he returned his gaze out the window. "She won't know anything until I come for her." He turned back toward Carlos. "How are my children?"

"They are fine, my friend. Healthy, fat, and smart. They will be excited to see you."

"Not as much as I will be to see them. And I expect that Benita's father still knows nothing."

"Nothing."

"He won't be so happy to see me once he learns."

"He's a loyalist. God help him, just like you used to be."

"Well... things change. And I wasn't a loyalist. I... we were happy just doing our jobs and serving our people." He turned to look out the window again. "Had I been a loyalist, I would have handed you over to MININT long ago."

Fidel Castro established MININT, or the Ministry of Interior, in June 1961, shortly after the failed invasion at the Bay of Pigs by Brigade 2506. Funded by the US and trained by the CIA, the brigade comprised exiled counter-revolutionary Cubans who wanted to overthrow and oust Castro, but Castro's armed forces quickly defeated the group in only two days. The victory strengthened Castro's position, and he shortly vowed publicly to the world that he was leading a Communist revolution. "I am a Marxist-Leninist and shall remain a Marxist-Leninist until the day I die." Controlling his people and those who would oppose him through fear, a long-known tactic of Lenin, became Castro's guiding principle. To accomplish this, a strong and ruthless force would be required. MININT was born and not only were they successful in their operation, but its leadership also has a longstanding reputation for being corrupt and unilaterally taking action to punish the Cuban people to maintain order

"Welcome to the resistance, my friend."

They rode in silence. As they entered the town and passed the hospital, the place where he had worked, met Benita, fell in love, and would eventually marry her in the emergency room, he wished he could go back to those days. But he knew it couldn't be.

They turned off the highway in the middle of town and, after a couple more turns, stopped in front of a tin-sided house. Carlos shut off the car. Alejandro saw Benita's father look out the window. "There's Fredrico," he said.

"Moment of truth, my friend. Be quick about it. Get the children packed so we can be on our way. We must be at Playa Maceo by midnight. The boat won't wait forever."

"I know. Hopefully, the old man won't make trouble. I don't want to hurt him."

"Just get going. The clock is ticking."

Alejandro stepped out of the car. Benita's father, Fredrico, was already standing at the door. He called out. "Who is it?"

As he approached, Alejandro, in little more than a whisper, said, "It is me, Fredrico. Alejandro."

"How did you get here?"

"It is a long story. Let's go inside."

On entering the house, Alejandro called out. "Lucia! Antonio! Come! I want to see my children."

The two emerged cautiously from a room in the back. At first, they didn't know what to think, but the familiarity quickly flooded their memory. Lucia, the oldest, yelled, "Papa!" And both the kids ran to their father, who had now gotten down on his knees. They hugged tightly and kissed. After a while, their father backed away. "Now, just stand there, so I can look at you."

They did with huge smiles.

"My, look at how you have grown." Until then, Alejandro didn't know how to measure the four years that he had been away. Now it all stood in front of him. "Lucia. You are a young woman now."

"I am thirteen."

"I know. I know. And look at my Antonio. You are a little man. Have you been taking care of grandpa?"

"Yes, papa. Yes. I am a big boy now. I'm almost eight."

"That's right, you have a birthday coming up. We will have to celebrate!"

"Papa... where is momma?" asked Lucia.

The second Alejandro heard the question, his genuine happiness and smile changed to one more reserved. In that instant, he realized his father-in-law should have asked the same question the second they saw each other. Unless... Fredrico knew more than he should. He looked up at his wife's father.

Fredrico said, “What are you doing here?”

Alejandro addressed his kids. “Now you two go back to your room. I’ll be there in a minute.”

“But where is momma, papa?” asked Antonio.

“She is still at work. We will talk about that later. Go on now. I need to talk to grandpa.”

When the kids were gone. Fredrico asked again, “What are you doing here?”

“I’ve come for the children. I am taking them with me. Once we are safe, I will then go for their mother.”

“I can’t let you do that.”

“But you will. I have a feeling that I don’t have a lot of time. Tell me. What do you know?”

“I know you are a deserter. You have left your post and disgraced your name and your country. Colonel Garcia from the Ministry told me. He came by two days ago.”

“So, MININT is looking for me?”

“Alejandro, how could you have been so stupid?”

“Shut up. I need to get the kids and go if we’re going to have a...”

The door flew open and three light green uniforms stormed the house and surrounded Alejandro. Shortly after, a large, well-decorated man in dark green slowly entered the room and took charge. “What do we have here?”

Alejandro said nothing as a look of defeat stretched across his face.

“Señor Fredrico, you did well. Gracias. Your country thanks you.”

Alejandro looked at his father-in-law. “What have you done?”

His wife’s father turned and walked away.

“He called as soon as the car arrived,” said the man in dark green. “As he was instructed. At least he is loyal to his country.”

Lucia and Antonio ran back into the room.

“What is going on, papa?” asked Antonio.

“It is nothing. Everything is fine. Go back into your room. I’ll be there in a minute.”

“But, papa,” said Lucia.

The man in dark green spoke to the children. "I am Colonel Garcia, and you will do as you are told, and don't come back out until I tell you to return."

As soon as the children left, Alejandro charged after the Colonel, but the soldiers held him back.

"Don't you ever speak to my children again!"

Colonel Garcia slowly walked over to Alejandro and said, "That is fine, Dr. Cabrera. You have nothing to worry about. Those children... they are no longer your concern."

Alejandro growled, "Bastardo." Then spit in the colonel's face.

The colonel never flinched. He calmly removed a handkerchief from his pocket and carefully wiped his face, then he ordered, "Take him away!"

Fredrico watched from the door as they loaded Alejandro and Carlos into the back of a truck. Before the colonel got into his car to follow, he turned and nodded in appreciation to his loyal citizen.

Fredrico did not acknowledge the gesture. He walked back into the house and collapsed on the sofa. He couldn't be sure of what fate awaited his son-in-law. Perhaps a long prison sentence. *If he could have only been more devoted*, he thought. Then his picture changed when two singular gunshots rang out from somewhere in the close distance.

The next morning, in a cemetery only a few blocks away, they found Alejandro and Carlos draped over two headstones. Dead. Shot in the back of the head, execution style.

Chapter Two

"Okay, big boy," said Sylvia Mason. "It's time to put on the blindfold."

"Really?" said Nigel with a hint of disbelief. "Isn't it bad enough you have all the window shades drawn shut?"

"I told you it was all a secret and a surprise. Now stop being such a wet blanket."

"Ugh." Nigel looked past Sylvia and addressed the pilot. "Hey, Cam. Do you know where we're going?"

Cam Derringer, friend, local Key West private investigator, and boat bum had volunteered to fly them to Sylvia's secret location to avoid the extensive layover they would have experienced catching a connecting flight out of Atlanta. When in Key West, if you're going just about anywhere, you will go to Atlanta first.

Cam said nothing, but slowly turned and let Nigel read his expression.

"Okay," said Nigel, "that was my one dumb question for the day."

Cam maintained his stare.

"Stop looking at me like that."

Then everything went dark. Sylvia stretched the blindfold across his eyes and tied it around the back of his head.

"Sheesh!"

"It's only temporary. Cam needs to land and refuel. Once we're back in the air, then I'll take off the blinder. Till then..."

She leaned in and gave him a soft kiss on the lips. When she pulled away, Nigel's lips remained puckered and moved around, looking for more.

"You're an idiot, Mr. Logan. That's what I love about you."

"Hey! I thought we had an understanding. No dropping of the 'L' word."

"And we do, but I mean it more in a *brotherly love* kind of way."

"Now you're getting kinky..."

She kissed him again.

"... and I like it."

From the cockpit, Cam spoke back and forth to the tower through his headset, then turned to his passengers. "For crying out loud. I'm about to puke in my lap up here. Act normal and buckle up. They've just cleared us to land."

Nigel and Sylvia Mason have a special relationship. They met just a few months earlier in Key West while Nigel did push-ups on the bar at the Green Parrot. He and another youngster named Tommy competed to raise money for POSH, Paws Often Steal Hearts, a huge Christmas holiday fundraiser for the local SPCA. It was an enormous success.

Sylvia is a powerful and successful real estate developer. Not to mention one of the wealthiest women in all the Keys. And luckily for Nigel, very single.

Nigel and Tommy pounded out the push-ups with beaded sweat and rippled muscles. All the while, Ms. Mason and her large gaggle of high-society ladies threw their money, or their husbands' money, down on the bar and cheered for their favorite horse. There was little difference between what happened at the Green Parrot that night and the Kentucky Derby itself, except instead of mint juleps, it was rum drinks and tequila. It was then that Sylvia Mason took a special shine to Nigel. But it wasn't until Nigel and Cam saved Christmas from certain disaster that her affections for him solidified. No. There would never be exclusive ties. That they agreed upon, but their bond was strong, and they would enjoy each other as long as the other could stand it. Which they both knew could be a week, or a lifetime.

Nigel and Sylvia remained on the plane as Cam handled the refueling. When he returned, shut the door, and climbed back into the cockpit, Nigel said, smiling, “We’re in Mexico. Ha!”

Cam and Sylvia exchanged glances. Of course, he was right, Cancun, but they didn’t have to admit it.

“What makes you say that, buddy?”

“I heard the guys on the ground speaking Spanish.”

“Wow,” said Cam, “you’re quite the investigator. Have you ever had a conversation with the ground crews in Texas, New Mexico, or Arizona, or Miami, for that matter?”

Nigel’s smile faded.

“That’s what I thought. So, sit tight and let me get this bird back in the air.” Then Sylvia can let you look around.

“You’ve become quite the smart ass lately, Cam.”

“I didn’t get this way naturally. Though some would disagree. I gained it as a learned skill. By hanging around with you! Once I get rid of y’all for a few days, maybe my nerves will settle and I can get back to normal.”

“You just did it again.”

“I know! Sylvia! Help me out here.”

She said, “I know how to shut him up.” Then she leaned over for a long, passionate kiss.

Cam rolled his eyes. “I don’t know what is worse. Listening to him chatter or hearing you two moaning and groaning. Buckle up. We’ll be taking off soon.”

Once they reached a comfortable cruising altitude, Sylvia unbuckled her and Nigel’s seatbelts and removed the blindfold. “Is that better?” she asked.

“Much.”

“I’m going to get me a drink. Do you want something?”

“The usual.”

She came back with a gin and tonic for herself and a Diet Coke for him. Then she sat in his lap and kissed him. She felt his lap respond, so she gave him a wink and a little wiggle. The smile on his face spoke volumes of mischievous thoughts, so she mouthed the word, *what*?

He wiggled his finger so he could whisper in her ear. She listened, then leaned back and slapped him on the arm. "You're awful. Awfully evil," she whispered.

He whispered back. "Ask me. Just make it loud enough for him to hear."

She couldn't stop giggling, but once she gained her composure, she nodded her head several times. *Okay. Okay*. Then she took a deep breath and said, "Hey, big boy... ever been a member of the mile-high club!"

Two seconds later, the headset came off, and Cam turned. "NOT ON MY PLANE!"

Nigel and Sylvia couldn't stop laughing.

Chapter Three

Cam landed, delivered the goods, refueled, and said his goodbyes and farewell wishes before heading off to return to Key West. Sylvia held Nigel by the elbow and guided him along as they stood in line, herded like cattle, waiting to clear immigration and customs.

"I think it's safe to say that you can take this silly thing off now," he said.

"Why do you say that?"

"Well, if I hear one more person say, 'Welcome to Belize,' I might be inclined to think we're in... I don't know... maybe Belize. Now take this thing off."

She did.

"Thank you."

"But we still have another puddle jumper to catch."

"And that blindfold can just stay in your purse. You've accomplished your goal. I am surprised. This should be nice. I've always wanted to visit, and now... here I am."

"Oh, darling. If you think you're surprised now, just wait."

Clearing customs only took about thirty minutes. An hour later, they were walking across the tarmac from the Maya Airlines terminal to the single turboprop Cessna that awaited them. The ground crew helped them aboard and they got comfortable.

"Placencia, huh?" asked Nigel. "I understand they have some of the best beaches in the world. Could it get any better?"

"Just wait, my dear."

"You're scaring me."

Moments later, the pilot and co-pilot boarded. "Are we ready to go?" The pilot asked with a smile and very good English.

Nigel looked around. The plane had seating for eight. He looked at Sylvia. "Are we the only ones on this bird?"

She gave a feigned look of surprise. "Well, I don't know. Seems to be the case."

Once they were in the air, the plane banked and headed due east. Nigel thought nothing of it until it was clear they were taking a detour. "Where are we going? Placencia is south of Belize City. Very south."

Again, she said, "Well, I don't know." But this time, her expression said something entirely different.

The plane descended toward the water and the copilot turned and said, "Look. It is the Turneffe Atoll."

The massive circular island was beautiful. From the air, it was stunning. The pilot made several long circles to improve their ability to see. The copilot asked, "You like it?"

"It is simply gorgeous," said Sylvia. "Breathtaking."

"Very good," said the copilot. "Next stop, Lighthouse Reef and the Great Blue Hole."

Nigel looked at Sylvia. "Oh, my, God. The Great Blue Hole... I've always wanted to see it. You arranged all this, didn't you?"

She answered with a smile, and he kissed her.

Lighthouse Reef creates the second of three atolls that exist off the waters of Belize. All of which offer some of the best snorkeling and diving in the Caribbean. Glover Reef being the third. They are equally beautiful, but only Lighthouse Reef has the Great Blue Hole. It's a near perfectly symmetrical sinkhole that had developed during several phases of the ice age when water levels were much lower. A popular diving location, it offers a variety of sea life and underwater caverns, complete with stalactites. It is almost one thousand feet wide and drops to a floor of over four hundred feet. In 2018, two submarines descended into the depths to map the hole's floor. They discovered two divers that had perished and settled on the floor. They reported the bodies to Belizean authorities, but out of respect, left them at their ultimate resting place.

From the air, the reef and hole were beautiful. The pilots made several banking rounds to provide a better view. When the plane leveled off and headed back toward the mainland, Nigel looked at Sylvia and said, "That was wonderful. It can't get much better than that."

"Oh, you silly man. I'm glad you enjoyed that, but I thought I taught you long ago not to underestimate me. There is plenty of daylight left and so much more to discover."

The landing at Placencia Airport was as smooth as any. But to call it an airport might be a stretch. The runway is just a little over twenty-one hundred feet and covers the entire width of the peninsula. At least it's paved.

Flying low over the water on the approach was exciting. Nigel and Sylvia both took a window seat for the landing. The lower and lower the plane flew, the more exciting it became. Then, just as it looked like the wheels would touch the water, land and pavement suddenly appeared, and they touched down.

A car was already waiting for them. As they approached, the driver got out smiling, opened the door, and they got in the back. Once he got behind the wheel, he said, "Ms. Mason, I presume?"

"That would be correct, and this is..."

"Mr. Logan, yes. We are expecting him as well. I hope you had an enjoyable flight from Belize City, yes?"

"Very much so. Thank you. How far is it to the marina?"

"Marina?" asked Nigel.

"You just hush. And enjoy the ride."

Nigel said nothing, but smiled.

"The marina is not far, and the boat leaves at three. We have plenty of time."

"The boat?" asked Nigel. "Where the hell are we going?"

Sylvia ignored Nigel and addressed the driver. "Very good. Ignore Mr. Logan. Right now, he is just tagging along." Then she addressed Nigel. "And, mister, if I have to tell you to hush one more time, I'll take that blindfold and use it as a gag."

Nigel leaned forward and spoke to the driver. "You see what I have to deal with here? She is as bossy as they come."

The driver laughed and spoke to Nigel through the rearview mirror. "I know what you mean, Mr. Logan. My girlfriend can be very bossy too, but I like the things she makes me do."

"Does it involve blindfolds?"

With a crooked grin, the driver said, "Sometimes."

Nigel flopped back in his seat and turned his head to catch Sylvia, biting her lower lip. "Okay, I give up," he said. "You win."

She gave him a long kiss, then pulled back just enough for them to see eye-to-eye. "I always do."

Five minutes later, the car pulled into the Wild Orchid Resort and the small private marina known as Orchid Raye. A dockhand took their small carry-on bags and said, "Follow me, please."

A single boat rested at the dock, triple 200 horsepower Yamaha engines hung off the stern. The boat's captain met them and took the bags from the dockhand, then offered a hand to Sylvia. "May I help you aboard, ma'am?"

After the skipper helped Sylvia, Nigel stood on the dock with a handout, waiting for assistance, but all he got was a roll of the eyes and a snickering smirk.

Nigel got aboard with a little fun huff. "Well, be that way then!"

With charged flutes of champagne, the boat eased out of the channel and toward open water. Sylvia made herself comfortable while Nigel roamed around to admire the vessel. He entered the cabin and found multiple copies of the same resort pamphlets scattered about. "Humph!" Then he went up to the flying bridge to join the captain. "Hey, skip. How long does it take to get there?"

"About an hour. Please, enjoy the ride."

"I will, thank you."

Nigel sat next to Sylvia. The deckhand came out with more champagne. Nigel refused, but Sylvia held out her glass.

"Ray Caye Resort, huh?"

"Yes! Aren't you surprised?"

"You bet. I'm surprised you would drag me out to some old decrepit, rundown, drag of a resort."

She slapped him. "I'm warning you. Behave... until I tell you otherwise."

Two staff members greeted them at the dock. One took their bags while the other handed them tall, colorful rum drinks. Then he tilted his head and gestured with his hand. “Right this way.”

Nigel and Sylvia were escorted throughout the island. The guide pointed out the Lionfish Bar & Grill. “We open for dinner at six thirty. But if you get hungry before then, just drop in and somebody will take care of you.”

They ended up at an oceanfront villa. The staff member opened the door and announced, “Your honeymoon suite awaits you.”

Nigel motioned for Sylvia to pass through first, and as she did, he uttered, “Honeymoon suite, huh?”

She turned back and winked.

He followed and said, “Did we take a trip to Vegas that I can’t seem to remember or something?”

After a short walkthrough of the villa, the staff member said, “My name is Miguel. If you need anything, just call. I hope you enjoy your stay with us here at Ray Caye.” Nigel held out a twenty-dollar bill, but Miguel declined. “Thank you, but no. Your best gratuity will be to have a splendid visit.” Then he was gone.

Nigel walked over to a window to watch Miguel leave and look around. He felt Sylvia’s arms slide around his waist to hug him from behind.

“Did you find anything strange about the walk over here?” he asked.

“No, honey. What do you mean?”

“It’s so quiet. And... and I can’t remember seeing anybody else. What about you?”

“No! And I better not while we are here.”

Nigel turned around in her arms to look at her. “What?”

“Nigel, the place is ours. Yours and mine, alone.”

“Ha! Well, I certainly hope so. Can’t imagine having to share this villa with some...”

“The entire island, you idiot. It is ours.” She held him tighter. “For three days, it is ours to enjoy, just you and me, and me and you, and you and me, and...” She kissed him and he kissed her back as they navigated through the villa to the single, king-size bed that faced an open sliding glass door, leading to a private swimming pool/spa, and the beautiful azure waters of the western Caribbean. She backed him up to the edge of the mattress and pushed him. He landed on his back and looked upon her with a grin as she unbuttoned her blouse.

"What other surprises do you have in store for me?" he asked.

She slipped off her blouse, unhooked her bra, let it all fall to the floor, and reached out a hand toward him. "I'm out of surprises today, Mr. Logan. I'm thinking it's your turn."

He grabbed her hand and pulled her down to join him.

Chapter Four

The next morning, Nigel rolled out of the sack as soon as his eyes opened. The red numbers on the digital clock read 3:07. He scrunched his eyes and thought, *I normally wake at four*. Then he remembered. Belize was on Central Time.

He wanted coffee, but the villa was nothing more than a big, elegant bedroom, with exceptional bathroom amenities and a stunning ocean view. There was no kitchen. All the dining and drinks could be obtained at the grill. Coffee, he had been told, was kept fresh twenty-four seven. He slipped into the bathroom to take a quick shower, taking care to be quiet. He didn't want to wake her. While she is typically an early riser too, he was quite confident that after yesterday's fun-filled and exciting travels, the pre-dinner sex, the fulfilling, fantastic cuisine from the grill, the late-night walk, the skinny-dip swim off the end of the pier, and finally the playful love making until they fell asleep in each other's arms, that she would sack it in a little longer than usual.

After his shower, he threw on some shorts and slipped out the door to head to the grill. He tasted the coffee. Yes. Fresh. He found a carafe, filled it, and returned to the villa, entering from the oceanfront. He sat by the pool and enjoyed his coffee. The sliding glass door was still open, and the mid-March springtime sea breeze felt cool to his skin. There was enough accent lighting in the villa that his night vision allowed him to see Sylvia sleeping comfortably. At some point, while he had been gone, she had curled herself into a bed sheet cocoon.

To the east, the sun warmed the horizon. As he admired her and his surroundings, he wondered how much this was costing her, but would never inquire. It would insult her to no end, yet the curiosity remained. And why splurge on him? While they very much enjoy each other's company, they also maintain their full independence. They weren't connected at the hip, nor did they want to be. She didn't demand things from him, and he reciprocated. Most men would want to exploit her wealth and latch on for all it's worth. After all, she is one of the most sought-after eligible catches in all the Keys. Any man would love to be in his shoes, but for more selfish desires. His interests didn't covet such, and she knew and appreciated it. Their relationship was affectionate, but more importantly, free of complications.

He got up and walked to the bed to sit and gaze at her. Her breathing was easy. A smile of innocence stretched across her face. *She's dreaming*, he thought. His thoughts of her brought an internal chuckle.

She had two sides. With an audience, she was serious, powerful, and confident. Bossy, but productive. Never insulting, or with an air of arrogance. However, when it was just the two of them, she became the girl next door. A sweet, humble lady eager to be held and loved. He liked both sides of her. He gently stroked her head, then got up for more coffee. As he walked back out toward the pool, the sun had marched even closer to the horizon. He filled his cup, took a sip, closed his eyes, and inhaled the scent of the sea.

When he opened his eyes, he felt the weight of Sylvia's fingers on his arm. She stood over him wearing her white chiffon shirt that didn't quite cover her bare butt, still unbuttoned from the night before. She crawled upon his lap, tucking her legs beneath her, stretching her arms around his neck, and kissed him behind the ear. "Good morning, honey," she said. "Did you get up at four again?"

"Good morning and yes, like always."

"What time is it now?"

Nigel looked out over the water. The sun was up above the water, but it hadn't been for long. "Does it matter? I figure the only *time* we need to be concerned with is checkout time."

She smiled. "I guess you are right."

"So, what would the Queen of Ray Caye like to do today?"

"Right now, this."

"And what about later?"

She shrugged. "Nothing. No agenda. I just want some quiet time with you."

"I'm good at doing nothing. It's probably one of the best things I'm known for."

She squeezed his neck, bit on his ear, and then said, "You, Mr. Logan, underestimate your many talents."

Later, as Nigel and Sylvia enjoyed breakfast at the grill and the sun warmed the Caribbean sky, another plane from Belize City descended and touched down on the runway of the Placencia airstrip. Two men dressed in tropical splendor got out of the plane and approached the taxi they had reserved. As a small pushback tug connected to the plane and moved it to a safe place on the apron to wait, the driver stood outside his door and asked, "Where to?"

"Placencia Medical Center," said one man.

Neither of the men smiled, but both looked distinguished. They were all business and on business. This wasn't a social call for pleasure. They were of medium build, fit, but not overly stocky. One wore a beige linen sport coat and matching slacks. His dark hair was kept short, while his ice-colored eyes stood in great contrast to his brown skin and heavy five o'clock shadow. The other one looked more buff, perhaps because he was clean-shaven, wore light shorts and a dark green guayabera shirt, a matching fedora, and aviator sunglasses.

As they arrived and the taxi stopped out front, the suit looked at his watch. Seven forty.

The driver turned toward their passengers. "They open at eight."

"Park over there," said the suit. "We'll wait."

As the taxi moved, two females walked around the corner to make their way toward the clinic. The fedora nudged his partner. "Cleto. Look. There she is. Should we..."

"No. We will wait. Making a scene outside would not be a good idea."

At ten after eight, Cleto patted the driver on the shoulder. "Wait here. We'll be right back."

"That's fine," said the driver. "The meter is running."

Cleto looked at his partner. "Let's go, Ramon."

The receptionist behind the counter looked up and saw the two men approach. Introductions were unnecessary. The two made quarterly trips, but this one came only two weeks after the last. It made the woman wonder. Despite the familiarity, both men flashed their identification, but the clinical worker already knew what they showed. La Embajada de Cuba.

The receptionist smiled. "How can we assist the embassy today?"

"We need to speak with her," said Ramon.

"She is with a patient. If you have a seat, I will tell her you are here."

Ramon looked at Cleto and motioned toward the lobby with his head.

Ten minutes later, Dr. Benita Cabrera came to the counter. The men noticed and approached, and despite her total disdain for the men, she maintained a professional deportment.

"Good morning. What can I help you with?"

"We need to speak in private," said Ramon.

"About?"

The two men looked at each other, then Cleto said, "When was the last time you heard from your husband?"

Benita gave a slight gasp, then gestured for them to come around the counter. "In my office, please."

She held the door as they entered. She sat behind her desk. "Please... have a seat."

They continued to stand. "This won't take long," said Ramon. "Again, when did you last communicate with your husband?"

"I received a letter from him, maybe a month ago. Why? What is this all about?"

"Do you still have the letter?" asked Cleto.

"Of course."

"We need to see it," demanded Ramon.

"Absolutely not. It is private."

Ramon and Cleto looked at each other. Ramon gave a nod and Cleto went behind the desk and grabbed the doctor by the neck. She reached up with both hands to pull his hand away, but couldn't.

"Where is it?" he said.

She shook her head, but he squeezed harder. Her eyes cut to Ramon when he said, "Give us the letter, or you will end up like Alejandro."

Ramon saw the dread in her eyes.

As Cleto squeezed harder, her hand found the drawer handle and pulled. She reached, grabbed a handful of papers and dropped them on her desk.

Cleto released her and shuffled through the various correspondences.

She held and rubbed her neck as she tried to catch her breath.

Cleto handed the letters to Ramon.

She coughed and uttered, "I'm sure... you already know what is in those letters."

Ramon looked up from the letter to gaze at her. Then he went back to reading.

She couldn't be sure, but based on the circumstances that she and her husband found themselves in, any mail sent to one another would be flagged and reviewed by the embassy before forwarding.

Terrified, she said, "Where is Alejandro?"

"Not in Venezuela," said Cleto.

"Callarse la boca! Shut up, Cleto."

Ramon tossed the letters down on the desk. "It would seem your husband has been idiotic, Ms. Cabrera."

She said nothing and listened.

Meanwhile, out at the front counter, the receptionist was ensuring patients that Dr. Cabrera would be with them shortly. Moments later, a wailing cry and moan came from her office. The receptionist ran to the door. She wanted to go in but knew that wouldn't be a good idea. As she stood there, the door opened, and the two men brushed by and headed to the front door. She watched them, and once they left the building, ran to the doctor.

Dr. Cabrera sat slumped over her desk, moaning and crying. "Dr. Cabrera... Ms. Benita, what is wrong?"

The doctor looked up. She was gasping, trying to catch her breath as she shook her head from side to side. Then she slapped her palm on the desk and yelled at the ceiling, "Nooo! Dear God! My Alejandroooo!"

Chapter Five

Their mini vacation on Ray Caye couldn't have been better. Sylvia and Nigel did what they wanted to do, when they wanted to do it. The staff pampered them to no end. Nigel was sure the island personnel enjoyed only having to meet the needs of two people on the entire island. And to tell the truth, the two of them weren't needy at all. It must have felt like a working vacation for them. However, when service was required, the staff hustled and busted their butts. In appreciation, with grace and kindness, Sylvia tipped generously. Only once did she get testy, and that was with Nigel.

It was on the second day. They were enjoying the beach, but when he pulled out his wallet to tip the towel-girl, Sylvia smacked his hand and scolded him. The towel girl grinned at the playful banter, and as Sylvia slipped a few bills into the girl's hand, she uttered, "Gabriela, he's simply impossible."

In her best broken English, Gabriela said, "Si. But he is good for Ms. Sylvia, yes?"

Sylvia motioned with her finger for Gabriela to come closer. When she did, Sylvia whispered something in her ear.

Nigel looked away with crossed arms and a huff.

Gabriela quickly straightened up with a blush, nodded in appreciation of the gratuity, and squealed and giggled as she scurried away.

Nigel turned toward Sylvia; arms still crossed. "What did you tell her?"

"That you think you are gay, but I've proved you wrong."

"Sheesh! And you call me impossible."

She sent him a wink. "Come on. Let's swim."

Mostly, except for that one moment of Sylvia's sassy fun, she was a vacation professional: calm, relaxed, carefree, and unapologetically loving. Never once did she call her office. And her staff, despite feeling the urgency to reach out to her because of developing difficulties, knew better than to disobey their only order. "Do not contact me under any circumstances. Period. Or look for other work." Once she returned, she would be up to her ass in alligators, and she expected it. Fear not, though, Sylvia and Nigel would return to Key West. The savvy businesswoman would once again surface and start grabbing bulls by the horns. Nigel would grin, back away, and give her all the space she needed. Despite their splendid time, he knew he would be her last thought, if any at all, in the coming days or weeks. He was fine with that. Business is business. It wouldn't be personal.

On the morning of their checkout, Nigel and Sylvia made the best of the time they had left on the island. They made sweet, tender love as the sun rose toward the sky. Then they curled themselves in the sheets and held each other. Nigel noticed a distant stare in her eyes, and he said nothing.

After a few minutes, looking out over the water, she said, "I'm going to miss this."

He leaned back to look at her better, but she wouldn't make eye contact. He could tell. She was shifting back to reality.

"Well, you know what they say, 'All good things must come to an end.'"

She turned to look up at him. "Who in the hell are *they*, and what in creation do they know?"

"I don't know. Some gaggle of old, bald, fat white guys that at one time thought they had all the answers."

She buried her face in his chest. "Screw them."

She pushed back to look at him. "Does it have to end?"

Nigel gazed into her eyes and said nothing.

She rolled over on her back. "I know, dammit."

"Come on. Stop it. We only have a few hours left. Let's go to the dock for one last swim to rinse off. Then we'll grab some breakfast."

She rolled back over toward him. "Sounds great, but make love to me first, like it might be the last time."

Nigel pulled them free of the sheet. "Why do you say that?"

"Because we never know. Do we? It's that way between us, right?"

Nigel felt his heart skip a quick beat, then said, "Yeah, I guess you're right."

"It's the way we wanted it, remember?"

Nigel nodded.

"A part of me hates that, but come here. Take me. All of me, and make sure I never forget it or you."

They finished in a drenching sweat, Nigel rolled onto his back, and they both panted and stared at the ceiling. Little smiles stretched across their faces. Sylvia broke the silence. "Okay, I think we really need to rinse off now." Nigel was still breathing hard but nodded his head.

Within thirty seconds of slipping into the beautiful, clear Caribbean water, Sylvia slipped out of her bikini. Nigel watched as she swung it around a few times before tossing it up on the dock. "It's a saltwater bath, right?"

Nigel followed suit and walked toward her. She tilted her head back in the water, letting her hair flow backward. She used her hands to smooth back her hair and said, "I'll scrub your back, if you'll scrub mine."

They were just off the end of the dock, rubbing and rinsing off every inch of skin when a gentle coughing noise interrupted them.

They looked up. It was Roberto, their normal morning server.

He rubbed his hands nervously, gazed adoringly upon Nigel, but spoke to Sylvia. "Good morning, miss. I saw y'all come to the dock." Then he placed the fingers of one hand on his chin and spoke over his fingertips. "I know you haven't had your coffee yet, so I brought you a carafe along with fresh towels."

Sylvia looked at Roberto, who had yet to take his eyes off Nigel. Then she looked at Nigel, who appeared to be oblivious to the attention he was getting. She gave a little giggle and Nigel looked at her.

"What?"

She motioned with her head toward Roberto and whispered, "I think someone might have a little crush on you."

"Huh? What?" He looked up at Roberto, who was back rubbing his hands together. Nigel always figured he was a little light in the loafers, but he had always been such a professional. Nigel looked back at Sylvia, who was grinning from ear to ear.

"He's just the sweetest thing," said Sylvia. "Be nice."

Nigel nodded his head, then turned his attention toward their server. "Roberto. I'm not sure what you have heard, but it would appear..." He gave Sylvia another glance. Then he continued, "I guess I've been wrong all this time."

Roberto put fingers to his cheeks. "Wrong about what?"

"Well, it seems I've been confused. I... I..."

Sylvia said, "He's trying to tell you he isn't gay."

"He's not? Gabriela thought..."

"Nope," said Nigel, "turns out I'm cured."

The look on Roberto's face told him he had said the wrong thing. "I mean, not that I was sick or anything... or that you are... or that anyone that..." He looked over at Sylvia. "I'm an idiot."

"So, Ms. Sylvia, he's not gay. Not even a teeny weenie bit?"

"Roberto, there is nothing teeny weenie about him, and that includes being gay."

Roberto looked at Nigel, who now felt compelled to cover his front side.

"Sorry, Roberto. But thanks for the coffee and towels. We'll be up in a few minutes for breakfast before we ship out."

Roberto nodded, returned to being the professional, top-notch server he was and walked away.

Sylvia was now laughing. "You should have seen the look on your face."

"Oh, shut up and come here. See what you caused."

She crept toward him, wrapped her arms around his neck, and legs around his waist. "Kiss me, you fool."

When they came up for air, Nigel said, "Thank you for all this. I've had a wonderful time."

"Think nothing of it. It's been my pleasure. Thank you for coming."

As he stood in the water with her wrapped around his torso, the outdoor speakers played the Kenny Chesney song, "Come Over."

She kissed him again and said, "Dance with me."

She clung tighter and closed her eyes as he drifted around the sandy bottom. After about two minutes into the song, he navigated over to a sandy patch where a typically docile creature loomed beneath the surface. Seconds later, she felt him violently jerk away and bellow in agony. "AAARGH! DAMMIT! ARRGH!"

"What is it, baby?"

He set her down. "ARRRGH! SON OF A BITCH IT HURTS!"

"What is it?" she asked in a panic.

"Stingray! It has to be. My right foot. Oh, shit, it hurts."

"Let's get you to the dock."

They did, and a very naked Sylvia and Nigel climbed the swim ladder. She went first and immediately saw the staff running their way to assist. Nigel could probably have been heard three islands over.

With every step of his right foot, Nigel clenched his teeth. Coming up the swim ladder was the worst. Putting pressure on his right foot felt like a spike driving through his foot and leg. He was no longer vocal about his pain except for the low growl.

On the dock, Nigel looked down at the inside of his right foot and saw the long-barbed stinger buried into his foot, and through his growling, uttered, "Sumbitch." He looked over at Sylvia. "I'm so sorry."

"Don't be silly." She looked up as the staff arrived. Roberto gave Sylvia a towel and covered Nigel.

In no time, they helped Nigel to a chair and produced a bucket of very hot water. They didn't have to tell him what to do. He immediately submerged his foot and slowly the hot water started to ease the pain. Once he could catch his breath, he looked at Sylvia and said, "When I lift my foot, grab that sucker and jerk it out."

"Are you kidding me?"

"No, I am not. It has to come out. I don't think I can do it myself." Sylvia had her towel wrapped around her body and shook her head, then looked at the faces of the staff that stood around. They were all shaking their heads, too. *Nope. Not me.*

The property manager finally arrived and placed a hand on Nigel's shoulder. "How are we doing? Let me look."

Nigel lifted his foot. "Yank the sucker out of there, dammit!"

"I'm afraid not." He looked over at Sylvia. "I'm sorry, but it appears you will check out a bit early. I will arrange a boat. He needs medical attention that we can't deliver. And again, I am sorry."

"It is fine. We had a splendid and wonderful time. Now, it will be more memorable than ever."

The pain wasn't completely gone, but it was manageable. Nigel tilted his head to look at Sylvia. "Not funny."

She ignored him. "I will go collect our things and meet y'all in the lobby."

"That will be fine," said the manager. "I have already sent for a wheelchair."

With a hint of playful sarcasm, Nigel said to the manager, "Do you mind if I get dressed before we leave?"

"If you wish."

"I think that might be a good idea."

Then Roberto crossed his arms and gave a little huff.

Chapter Six

With no means to keep the water hot enough during the boat ride back to the mainland, the discomfort, then pain, slowly returned. The barbed stinger that remained protruding from the side of his foot was painful enough on its own, but as the water cooled, the pain caused by the stinger's release of a complex venom made matters worse.

As the pain slowly crept back, Nigel kept his eyes closed and tried to remain focused. The incident brought forward memories of a past, but brief, lover by the name of Emma Baxter. They had met under similar circumstances. Nigel had been going through a rough and difficult time. And, after waking up on the beach amongst empty beer cans, a nearly empty bottle of bourbon, and a huge hangover, he rushed to Emma's need when she too collected a snapped-off stingray barb in her foot. Emma was brave. She refused medical treatment, and, while under the foggy influence of Jim Beam, it was up to Nigel to remove the stinger.

She was going through a difficult time as well. Luckily, her troubles were of the nature in which Nigel's special talents could intervene and resolve the ugly issue. In the end, their relationship grew into an affectionate bond that had more to do with healing each other than sex. They were there for each other when they needed it most.

At that moment on the boat, he missed her company. She would have jerked that barb from his foot, if for no other reason than to pay him back for the pain he had caused her when he did the same. The thought brought a thin grin across his face.

"What has you in such a fine mood?" asked Sylvia. "I thought you were in pain."

Nigel opened his eyes and turned his head to look at her. "I am. Please find out if this tub has any whiskey on it. Preferably Jim Beam."

"You want booze? I didn't think you..."

"What? Drink anymore? No, I don't. Rarely anyway, but yes. I need something to take the edge off and I don't think there is enough Diet Coke in the world to do the trick."

She returned a couple of minutes later with a bottle of rum. "Here. This will have to do." She rolled her eyes. "The skipper says we're about fifteen minutes out."

Nigel took the bottle, read the label, and wanted to laugh, but the barbed stinger wouldn't have any of it. He took off the cap and took a long pull.

"Enjoy it while you can," she said. "They are the biggest titties I have to offer."

Nigel felt the warmth hit his belly. He took another sip, then looked at the label again. Big Titty 44 Double D Rum. "This stuff is excellent. It's big on flavor." He took another pull.

She glared at him.

Then he swallowed a mouthful, and with the enthusiasm of a fire-breathing dragon said, "But... I like your little perky ones better!"

"Smart answer, pal. Now let me see that bottle."

She took a good swig when he handed it over.

The same car and driver that brought them to the docks waited at the curb. As the skipper and the boat staff helped Nigel to the car, the driver ran around and opened the rear door. He said, "That's a nasty one for sure."

Nigel winced as they folded him into the back seat. "Any idea what kind of ray?"

"By the size of the stinger," said the driver, "I'd say a Southern. They get quite large, and the size of that stinger tells me it was no baby."

Sylvia joined Nigel on the other side, and the driver got behind the wheel.

"Where are we headed?" asked Sylvia.

"Placencia Medical Clinic. It is better than the hospital, and it isn't far. Dr. Cabrera is quite good, and she is very nice and pleasant."

Nigel tilted his head back on the backrest, tried to focus away from the pain, and said, "We'll see how nice she is when she removes this thing. Let's go. I'm ready for this part of the vacation to be over." Then he turned his head to look at Sylvia. With the best smile he could offer, said, "It's been fantastic until now. Thank you. Did you bring those big titties?"

She produced the bottle from her travel bag. "You're impossible. You know that, right?"

Before taking another good pull, he said, "It's my most endearing quality."

When he swallowed, she leaned over, kissed him on the lips, and enjoyed the remaining heat and aroma of the rum. As she pulled her lips away, she said, "I could argue otherwise." Then she went in for another kiss.

The driver watched them in the rearview mirror and smiled.

Sylvia broke away from their backseat affections when she felt the brakes and the slow turn into a parking lot.

Nigel took one last strong drink from the bottle. It burned the back of his throat and topped off the nice shine he had been working on. As they hobbled to the clinic, the receptionist came from around the desk to hold open the door. As they passed through, the driver looked at her and said, "Americanos."

The receptionist spoke very little English, but the sight of the stingray barb protruding from the side of his foot needed no translation. She ran for a nurse.

As they sat down, Nigel scanned the room. Four elderly people waited: one man and three women. He looked at the closest woman with one eye closed and pointed to his foot. "Stiiiingray."

She replied in Spanish. He couldn't understand a word, but nodded his head anyway, like he did. When she finished, he said, "That's what I was thinking."

A pretty nurse came out from the back. Maria on her nametag. "What have we got here?" Her English was very good.

Nigel lifted his foot. "Just a little sumpin, sumpin."

“I see. How bad does it hurt?”

Nigel gave her a wink. “I can’t remember.”

Maria looked at Sylvia.

“He’s self-medicated... on Big Titty.”

Maria smiled, looked at the receptionist, and said something in Spanish. She left and quickly returned with a wheelchair.

The nurse looked at Sylvia. “We will need some identification and information. Payment? Insurance?”

“Cash,” said Sylvia.

They transferred him into the chair, and the nurse pushed him. As she did, she spoke to the other patients in Spanish to apologize for making him a priority.

Nigel picked up on the word *prioridad*, looked back toward the waiting room, and said, “Sorry, Y’all.”

The nurse put him into a room, and he waited while Sylvia, along with the help of another English-speaking person, worked on the paperwork.

After a brief wait, a woman wearing a white lab coat and stethoscope around her neck entered the room. The conventional signature of *The Doctor*. Not to mention her name and title were embroidered on her coat. Benita Cabrera, MD. She looked upon Nigel with a level and manner of seriousness that took away some of the shine. She pulled gloves from a container, put them on, and went straight to her examination without saying a word. To Nigel, she was as attractive as any Latin American female he’d ever seen, except for the smile. She didn’t have one. Her expression told a story of busy anger, but not necessarily toward him.

As she gently prodded around the shaft of the barbed stinger, Nigel winced and sucked the pain back through his teeth. When she stood and took off her gloves, he said, “Where is the doctor I was told about? The nice and pleasant one.”

She ignored him and stoically said, “It is deep. It needs to be surgically removed.” Her English was also excellent.

Alcohol can make you say the dumbest things. “Can’t you just numb it up and jerk it out? With your demeanor, it seems you might enjoy that.”

Then the signs of her anger broke, and she spun away to sob. Sometimes anger and sadness run together as an emotional package, like a pack of dogs, wild and unpredictable.

Her reaction was sobering, and Nigel felt like an ass. "Doctor. I am so sorry. Please, forgive me."

She remained facing away, but she shook her head. "No, it is not you that needs to be sorry. It is me. Please forgive my bedside manner. I didn't mean to make you feel uncomfortable. I am not normally like this."

"May I ask how you normally are?"

She walked over to a table by the wall, pulled two tissues, and blew her nose. Then she turned around with a feigned smile that gave him a reflection of her usual self. "No, you may not. I'll send in a nurse to clean and prep the wound for surgery. Stay put."

Nigel lifted his foot. "Don't worry, Doc. Not going anywhere."

She smiled back, more genuinely than before.

Maria came back in. She gave him another basin of hot water, which helped knock off what remained of the pain from the venom. The site of the injury was another matter.

After letting it soak for a while, she lifted his foot and gently scrubbed around the protrusion with an antiseptic. She was careful not to add unnecessary pain but still cleaned the area well.

Now and then, she would hit the area just right and Nigel would flinch. She apologized every time. "I'm sorry."

"It's okay. May I ask you something, Maria?"

"Sure."

"The doctor seems very unhappy. I was a stupid wise-ass and made her cry."

"Yes. She is very sad. They buried her husband today."

Nigel closed his eyes tight. "Now I feel like an absolute jerk." As he shook his head in self-disappointment, her words sank into his numbed gray matter. "You said *they* buried him. And this was today?"

"Yes."

"Why is she here? For crying out loud."

"I don't know," she lied. "She must work."

The word *they* kept seeping in. "You said, '*They* buried him,' not she buried him. Did she not attend the funeral?"

The look on Maria's face answered the question without uttering a word.

"I've said too much," she said. "Forget it."

"Where did *they* bury him?"

"No. Please. Forget I said anything. I'll let Dr. Cabrera know that you're ready."

As she walked toward the door, Nigel said, "Where, Maria? I promise not to say a thing."

Maria stopped and held the doorknob. Without turning around, she said, "Our homeland... Cuba."

A little later, Sylvia joined him in the examination room with a smile, saying, "Never a dull moment, huh?" She saw the look on his face, said nothing more, and pulled a chair close to sit.

He reached for her hand. "Did you get everything settled?"

"Sure. Americano cash is king, even more so in Belize."

"Thanks."

"What's the matter?"

"I don't know. Something isn't right..."

He went on and told her what he knew.

"Sylvia, it doesn't make any sense, does it? You lose your spouse, and you don't even return home to attend his funeral."

"Maybe it wasn't a good marriage."

"No. I don't buy that. Like I said, 'Something isn't right.' She is clearly hurting. It is so sad."

Dr. Cabrera returned with Maria, doing her best to put on her best face. It wasn't working. As Maria washed her hands in the sink, the doctor said, "We will use a local anesthesia to numb the area. Maria will assist as I open the wound enough to extract the barb."

Nigel nodded. "Do what you have to do."

After washing up and putting on gloves, the doctor drew a sizable amount of Lidocaine into a syringe. When she sat at the foot of the table, she looked up at him and said, "This is going to burn at first."

Nigel nodded, then watched and winced as the needle moved around the wound site.

Sylvia turned away. "I can't believe you can sit there and watch that."

Dr. Cabrera finished, looked up with a smile, and said, "You did very well. As we wait for it to take effect, Maria will get you a sucker for being so brave."

Sylvia turned back around.

"Rum flavored?" asked Nigel.

"Grape, cherry, or root beer," said Maria.

"Make it a root beer, then."

As Nigel popped the sucker in his mouth, the doctor took the syringe needle and poked around the wound. "Feel anything, Mr. Logan."

"Nope! And call me, Chief."

"Okay, Chief, let's get started." She looked at Maria. "Number ten scalpel, please."

As the doctor held up the instrument, Nigel looked at Sylvia. Her eyes were glued to his foot. She didn't look good. "Are you going to be alright?"

The doctor looked up and saw the same ashy coloring on her face. "Ma'am, perhaps you should have a seat."

Sylvia nodded her head and wearily sat.

Nigel and the doc exchanged glances, and he added a little wink. He watched as she went back to work. Once she had enough tissue cut away from either side of the barb, she inserted a pair of straight hemostats alongside the stinger and backed it out. She held it up for Nigel to see. "I'm impressed. This is a big one."

Thump!

Nigel turned his head, and the doctor craned her head to look. Sylvia had passed out and fallen out of her chair. Maria dashed to check on her. After giving her a once over, she looked up. "She is fine. Maybe a headache later."

"Go get somebody to help you. Take her to the sofa in my office."

She did, and in less than a minute, Nigel and Dr. Cabrera were alone. With the stinger removed and the Lidocaine still working, she aggressively scrubbed the wound and prepared to close it. As she worked, Nigel said, "Sorry about Ms. Sylvia. I guess she's a little squeamish."

"It is fine. Don't worry about it."

"And..." he paused long enough for her to look up. "I'm sorry to hear of your husband's passing."

She looked away for a few seconds, then returned to his stare. "Maria shouldn't have said anything."

"Don't blame her. I pressed her for an explanation. And... I'm sorry for upsetting you earlier. That was uncalled for. I've been drinking. It's not a good one, but it's my only excuse."

She put on a thin smile and said nothing.

"When did he pass?"

"A few days ago."

"And his name?"

Tears flooded her eyes and streamed down her face. "Alejandro." She turned away and sobbed uncontrollably.

Nigel said nothing.

After a few beats, she stood, took off her gloves, and walked back to the sink. She washed her face and hands and pulled herself together. When she turned for another pair of gloves, she said, "Please, Mr. Logan. No more questions. I need to finish with your care."

Nigel nodded, and she returned to his needs. After closing the wound and bandaging it, she found a crutch for him to lean on. "You'll be good as new soon. How long are you in Belize?"

"We leave today."

"Then I expect you have a doctor back in the States to follow up with?"

"Yes."

Nothing was said for a spell, then Nigel said, "I can tell. You loved him dearly. He must have been a good man."

She nodded her head as the tears returned.

"Again," he said. "I'm very sorry for your loss."

She nodded more, and he headed toward the door. He stopped when she angrily said, "If he had only stayed in Venezuela."

As Nigel turned to look at her, Maria opened the door and saw the doctor's tears. Nigel looked at Maria. He held up a hand, and she backed out of the room. Nigel returned his focus to the doctor, gave her time, and then asked, "Would you like to talk about it?"

"You are a stranger. Why should I talk to you?"

"Maybe because I am a stranger. And sometimes a stranger, one that you will never see again, is the perfect person to lean on. Plus, you appear to want to talk about it."

She said nothing.

"Doc, can I call you Benita?"

She nodded.

"Good. And remember to call me Chief. Now, Benita, why didn't you… or couldn't you attend your own husband's funeral? Why are you even here working, of all days?"

"It is complicated."

"So am I, so give me a chance to understand."

"I serve as a member of the Henry Reeve Medical Brigade. It is a team of Cuban medical professionals that serve around the globe where there is a need for medical care."

"Okay, so what has that got to do with anything?"

"It is part of my contract to remain and work all my scheduled days."

"Why would you ever sign such a restrictive contract?"

"Again, it's complicated. I can't say any more."

"You mentioned Venezuela."

"I'm sorry. No. I've said enough. Please go. I have other patients."

Nigel watched as she turned and went out the door. Maria immediately came in with a wheelchair. Nigel eased himself back down. "How is Ms. Sylvia?"

"Very embarrassed."

Nigel wrinkled his nose.

"What is wrong?"

"I'll never hear the end of it."

Chapter Seven

Nigel was wrong. She said very little on the ride to the airstrip and during the flight back to Belize City. And since she again chartered the entire plane, the staff, pilot, and aircrew looked the other way when she boarded with the bottle of Big Titties in hand.

After takeoff and reaching their cruising altitude, Nigel asked, "Are you mad at me or something?"

She kept her head looking forward. "No, darling. Don't be silly."

"Well, you certainly could have fooled me by the way you are bogarting that bottle of rum."

Without looking, she reached out with the bottle.

He took it and laughed to himself. It was empty. "Thank you."

With her eyes closed, she offered a cool and soft, "You're welcome."

"Listen. While you were... ahhh... not in the room. I spoke to Dr. Cabrera. It was all so weird. I guess her husband had been in Venezuela. It sounded like he left and that, somehow, had something to do with his untimely death. Anyway, she said she was a part of this Henry something-something medical brigade, and she couldn't go back to Cuba for the funeral because her contract forbade it. I gently pressed for more details, but she got upset and left the room. Doesn't that just sound crazy, cruel, and unreasonable?"

Sylvia said nothing.

"Sylvia... Did you hear what I said?"

Still nothing.

Nigel leaned in and caught the light vibrato of her soft palate vibrating. She was asleep.

"Well, shit." He looked up and found the eyes of their stewardess in her jump seat. She smiled back, and he said, "Diet Coke, please."

She reached down into a cooler and tossed him a can.

Sylvia's and Nigel's eyes opened with the first squeal of tires on the runway. It startled her, and she reached and grabbed his arm. Nigel put his hand on her clenched fingers and said, "Easy now. It's okay. Boots on the ground."

She rubbed her eyes with her free hand, then looked at him.

"Good morning," he said. "You slept hard. Even if it was only for fifteen minutes."

"Did you doze?"

"I tried. The throbbing in my foot had other plans."

"You should have taken those painkillers the doctor prescribed."

"No need. I'll be fine with the Ibuprofen."

She hugged him. "You're such a silly, tough guy."

"Tough enough, I guess. You seem to be in a better mood."

She broke her embrace and went for her phone. "I have no idea what you are talking about."

At that moment, any idea of discussing her passing out cold in the doctor's office dissolved into the past.

Two seconds after taking her phone off airplane mode, it dinged with a text notification. She read the message.

Your chariot awaits.

She looked at Nigel. "It's Cam. He's here already."

"Good. I'm ready to get back to check on my boat."

Nigel lives on his sailboat, *MisChief*. She is a classic 1966 Pearson Vanguard, a cozy thirty-two-footer, and one of the prettiest girls at the dance. The perfect size for a minimalist like Nigel and the occasional overnight companion. He keeps her at the marina on the Naval Air Station, Key West, on Boca Chica Key.

It has almost been a year since he arrived there from his home in Port St. Joe, the quaint little coastal town on Florida's Forgotten Coast. He missed his friends and the town, but wasn't ready to return and pick up where he left off. He still felt he had some personal issues that needed to be sorted out. If that were even possible.

When Nigel first met Sylvia, the one thing she liked to complain about was his lack of proper transportation. He had a boat and an old Bronco, but the Ford was still in St. Joe. So, he had no car in the Keys, unless you considered his usual Uber driver that would pick him up at the front gate.

Truth was, he needed something. If he couldn't find a ride from the marina, the front gate made for a good, long walk. One day, he bit the bullet. He called her up. "Finally got me some wheels. What do you say I pick you up for a ride and some lunch? We could grab a late lunch at Louie's Backyard."

"Well, you old stubborn salt. I finally broke you. Do tell. What did you get?"

"It's a surprise."

"Oh! How do you know me so well? I love surprises. But please, one little hint."

"It's a Pedego."

"Oooo! Sounds sporty and Italian. Pick me up at... say, one-thirty?"

"It's a date. See ya then."

When he got to her house, he pressed the intercom button outside the gate. He didn't have to say anything. "Be out in a flash!"

As the gate parted, she saw him standing in the middle of the drive. She rushed to him and gave him a kiss. "Okay, big boy. Where is it?"

Nigel pointed over toward the side. She looked and found a red, built-for-two bicycle leaning up against the shrubs. Her brow came together, and her eyes brought to a slit. "Really?"

"Well, yeah. If you will remember, it was your idea."

"My idea?"

It was true, though she would never admit it, she once made a passing joke suggesting, "Get a bicycle built for two, or something for crying out loud."

"I can't be seen riding around town on that."

"Yes, you can, and yes, you will. Besides, it will be the coolest tandem bike in town."

"Why's that?"

"Because it's electric."

"You mean I don't have to pedal?"

"I never said that. Now get your ass on the seat!"

After clearing customs and immigration, they headed toward the terminal where Cam was waiting. She strolled along, and he hobbled on the crutch, keeping the weight off his foot. Suddenly, Sylvia stopped and spun Nigel around. She bounced up and kissed him on the cheek. "Thank you," she said. "I had a wonderful time."

"I should thank you. You're the one that picked up the tab."

"Oh, that was nothing. Besides, had I come down here alone or with anybody else, it would have been dreadful. You made the trip special."

Nothing, yeah right, he thought. He would never insult her by mentioning it but did a little research and found out their little exclusive island retreat came in at a hefty sixty thousand dollars, twenty grand a day before tips, other side gratuities, and transportation.

"Special, huh." Lifting his foot, he continued, "What about this?"

"Oh, darling. That alone was worth the price of admission."

He leaned over for a long kiss, and she gave him one. Then, from a distance, they heard an announcement. "Hey, lovebirds." They broke apart and looked toward the voice. It was Cam, using his hands as a megaphone. "Boarding time is over. Once the doors close, nobody else will be allowed on the plane. So, knock that crap off and get your butts in gear."

Nigel said, "He can be so damn pushy sometimes."

"He's your friend."

"I know. I know. Dammit."

Chapter Eight

Nigel sat up front with Cam. Sylvia got comfortable in the back and found it necessary to sleep off the rest of her morning rum. The ride home was a mirror operation to the trip down. Only one difference. No blindfold.

Through his headset, Nigel heard Cam ask, "So I gather you had a good time? She told me she reserved the entire island. I checked it out online. Impressive."

"It was wonderful until this morning. It was all great. Even the stingray gave me something to remember it by."

"I guess so. Does it still hurt?"

"Yeah, but nothing like when it happened. I've heard people describe how it feels, but my experience tells me they underplayed the pain. That will teach me not to shuffle my feet."

"And you say the stinger was how long?"

Nigel took his thumb and index finger and spread them apart as an illustration.

Cam shook his head and shoulders with the willies. "And how deep was it?"

Nigel squeezed his finger and thumb together less than half the distance.

"Damn," mumbled Cam.

They flew in silence for a long while until Cam noticed Nigel's deadpan stare out the window. "What cha thinkin' about?"

Nigel turned to look at his friend. "Ah, nothing really. Just replaying in my head scenes at the doctor's office."

"Let me call some bullshit on the, *nothing really* part. I've seen that look before."

Nigel said nothing.

"Want to talk about it?"

"Not really..."

But he did anyway and told Cam what he knew about the doctor who took such great care of him. "It was all so sad and disturbing."

"That's more than sad?" said Cam. "That's just wrong."

"She was so upset," said Nigel, "and deservingly so, yet she still took care of me like a pro. I wish..."

"You wish what? It isn't like you can do anything about it."

"I know. It's just..." Nigel turned his head to stare out the window again.

"Hmm," grunted Cam. "She's pretty, isn't she?"

"Gorgeous," said Nigel to the outside world.

"Uh, huh..."

Nigel turned his head. "What?"

Cam said nothing and gave a stare.

"Oh, stop it. Like you said, there isn't anything we can do."

"We? What's this *we* stuff? You got a rat in your pocket?"

"Just fly your plane, will ya?"

After a few minutes, Nigel said, "By the way... thanks for doing this. We appreciate it."

Cam smiled, then looked back toward a sleeping Sylvia before returning his attention toward Nigel. "Trust me. I'm being well compensated."

"I'm not surprised. She's a mess, isn't she?"

"You'd know better than me, brother."

On their final approach, Cam spoke into his headset. "Ladies and goons, the seatbelt light is on. Make sure your seats and tables are in an upright position and prepare to land."

Sylvia, now wide awake, spoke into her headset. "You're a nut, Cam. But you got the *goon* part right."

Nigel slowly turned around to look at Sylvia. She returned his stare by sticking out her tongue.

Cam landed at EYW, Key West International, with the gentle ease of a professional, slowed, turned around, and taxied back to his hangar. Once they were outside the aircraft, Sylvia turned her phone on and it exploded with text notifications. Her staff had been given strict orders not to disturb her on the trip, but that was then, and now was now.

"For crying out loud," she said. She glanced and read through a few messages. "You'd think I could escape for a few days and not come back to a shitshow. Let's clear customs. I need to get to the office."

Cam said, "Hey, you two. Why don't y'all drop by the boat later for Wild Turkey cocktails with me and Diane?" Diane is his surrogate, unofficial adopted daughter.

Nigel looked at Sylvia, who hadn't heard a word Cam said. She was firmly back, lost in her professional chaos.

"Thanks," said Nigel. "But I think we'll take a raincheck. Give our best to Diane."

"Will do."

When they cleared and were walking/hobbling out of the airport, Sylvia unapologetically said, "I need for you to take an Uber back to the base. I'm up to my ass in problems, but what's new? Take care."

Nigel watched as she walked away. "Hey," he called after her. "Not even a little goodbye kiss?"

She stopped and turned around with a little huff. Then dashed back to him and kissed him on the cheek. "Aren't you a needy one?" Then she turned and was off again.

With a smile, he said, "Call you later!" But she was already on the phone, barking orders and making demands. The smart, savvy, and demanding Sylvia was back in full mode. God, help them.

Teddy, Nigel's Uber driver, dropped him off at the gate. The gate guard went inside the shack and returned with Nigel's bike. "Damn, Chief. This thing sure takes up a bunch of space." As he wheeled it out to the pavement, he saw the bandaged foot. "What happened?"

"Long, stupid story. Thanks for keeping my bike safe and take this." Nigel held out the crutch. "Find a dumpster for it, please."

"No problem."

Nigel mounted his big bike. With the condition of his foot, there would be little to no pedaling. But that was okay. He powered up the unit, twisted the throttle, and was off to the marina.

Chapter Nine

It was now early April, and Nigel's injury was much better. The wound showed a little redness. There wasn't enough tenderness when he walked to cause a limp, but enough to remind him of the incident. As he walked into Navigator's, the marina bar, he reminded himself. *Shuffle, Shuffle, Shuffle… Always shuffle.* Nigel grabbed stool seventeen, and, from the far end of the bar, the manager slung a can of Diet down toward the other end. Nigel grabbed it. "Thanks, Steve."

Steve was polishing glasses as he eased down the bar. As he drew close, Nigel looked around the room. "Slow day, huh?"

"It's Monday, Nigel. And I just opened a few minutes ago. Plus, after last night, I'm sure the regulars are still licking their wounds. Speaking of which, how is your foot coming along?"

"Gets better and better every day. In a minute, I'm going into town to have the stitches removed."

"Why not do it yourself?"

"I guess I could." Nigel flung his flip-flop and foot on the bar.

"Not here, dammit," barked Steve.

Nigel laughed. "I'll see ya later. Gotta run before the clinic closes. Thanks for the DC. Put it on my tab."

His appointment was at 1715, the last slot of the day. It was with a PA, a physician's assistant named Juan Cruz at a little private clinic on Eaton Street that had once been a private residence. Teddy, Nigel's favorite Uber driver, dropped him off fifteen minutes early as requested to fill out paperwork. Knowing how a doctor's office can be, he expected to have to wait. Then a door opened, and his name was called. Nigel looked at this watch: 1717. He smiled at the nurse.

"Right this way," she said.

She led him to an examination room, took his vitals, and documented the reason for his visit. When she slid her clipboard under her arm, she said, "Get comfortable. The physician's assistant will be in momentarily."

Two minutes later, there was a knock on the door. It opened.

The PA stuck his head inside the door. "Mr. Logan, I presume."

"Call me, Chief."

"Chief it is."

The PA came in and took a seat to make small talk about Nigel's visit. He was handsome and fit. Maybe six feet tall, one seventy-five to one-eighty. His baby-faced youthfulness might raise questions as to his qualifications. He looked like he was fresh out of high school, but his professionalism spoke volumes.

"So, Chief... I understand we have some sutures to remove. Tell me what happened?"

Nigel gave him the Reader's Digest version of his trip with Sylvia, making sure not to mention her name. There was no need to, except for bragging rights, and Nigel wasn't into that sort of thing. He told the PA about his misfortune with the monster stingray, the impaled stinger, and the excellent care he received in Placencia.

"That's the gist of it, doc. So, here I am."

"Belize is exquisite. My family is from Honduras, so I am very familiar." The PA rose, extended the end of the examination table, and went to the sink to wash his hands. "What do you say we take a look?"

Nigel sat back, shook off his flip-flop, and rested his foot on the extension. The PA sat back down, rolled his chair over, and carefully removed the bandage. "Ahhh, you did an excellent job of keeping it clean. Minimal redness and inflammation. Looks great. The doctor down there did a wonderful job."

Nigel watched as his PA put on gloves and went to work, snipping, pulling, and dropping the sutures in a basin.

"She's Cuban. Very kind and efficient." Nigel didn't feel the need to explain her predicament, but said, "She is part of some medical brigade or something. A Henry something maybe."

The PA stopped and looked up at Nigel, his expression not as pleasant as before.

"The Henry Reeve Medical Brigade?"

Nigel snapped his finger. "That's the one."

The PA's smile was no longer available, and he went back to his work.

"What's the matter, Doc?"

"Nothing." He lied. "I've heard of the organization." He continued to work as he spoke. "They once came to my homeland to provide medical assistance after hurricanes Eta and Iota made landfall in Nicaragua. Honduras was heavily affected, and the Henry Reeve brigade came to assist. Their doctors and nurses are excellent. I now understand how you received such excellent care." *Clink. Clink.* He dropped his scissors and tweezers in the metal basin. "We are all done, Chief. I would take it easy for a couple more weeks. After that, you should be good to go."

"Doc, before I mentioned the Henry Reeve thing, we seemed to get along just fine, but..."

The PA put on a forced smile. "But nothing. I am sorry. I was thinking of my people after the hurricane," he lied again. "As I said, the brigade has excellent doctors. You should feel fortunate that she took such good care of you."

"Oh, I do. Trust me."

"Have a wonderful evening, Chief. I must finish up today's paperwork and go home. Tomorrow will be another long day." With that, he left the exam room.

Nigel walked out to the front porch of the clinic. A rooster perched on one railing and a sleeping iguana rested on another. As he descended the porch stairs to the sidewalk, he almost called Teddy for a ride. Instead, he walked to the post office on Whitehead to check his box. It had been a while since clearing it out. When he opened the box, it was clear it had been more than just *a while*. It was crammed full. He took his parcel of envelopes and sale papers to a table to cull through them. Junk mail went into the circular file, and the potential meaningful mail got put into a separate smaller pile, if you could call two envelopes a pile.

Nigel looked at the first letter. It was a card from his buddy, Red, in Port St. Joe. He opened it. It was a simple card that read, *Miss you, brother*. Inside the card was a picture of Red on the beach with his net and a pile of mullet in the sand. *You old bastard*, he thought with a smile. "Miss you, too," he said aloud. Then he grabbed the second, more official-looking envelope. It was from the Placencia Medical Clinic. With scrunched eyebrows, he opened it. It was a bill for one hundred fifty-seven dollars, a note of apology, and a return envelope. They had undercharged him for his visit. He chuckled. At least he would get to pay for something for his painful vacation. Before standing in the post office line and getting a money order to mail back, he took a picture of the bill and texted it to Sylvia with a note: *What the hell!?!*

A couple of blocks later, Nigel strolled into the Green Parrot and mounted his stool. Travis, the bartender, eased down the line toward him. "Diet Coke?"

"Yeah, but add a splash of some Big Titties."

"Huh?"

"Big Titties... do you have any?"

Travis looked down at his chest. "I don't, but Tina will start her shift around eight."

Nigel shook his head. "Forget it. Just add some Cruzan and a lime."

"Whoa! You mean you want..."

"I don't want to hear it. I just want one. And only one. After that, I'll stick to the potent stuff."

Travis put Nigel's drink in front of him and asked, "How's the foot?"

"It's fine... but wait... who told you about that?"

"Derringer and Diane were in here last week. Said you tangled with a ray or something."

"What else did he tell you?"

"Nothing really. I just mentioned that I hadn't seen you. He said you were mending a bad foot. Why?"

"And he said nothing else? About how or where?"

"No. It was a ray right, so it had to have happened out at the beach or somewhere. Why would that be important?"

"It isn't. I was just... just forget it."

Nigel felt a little stupid. He knew Cam could and would keep a secret. It was silly of him to think he would go around yapping about his and Sylvia's adventures.

He took a sip of his rum and diet. It was tasty. Then his phone rang. He looked at the screen and smiled.

"Well... hello Ms. Mason," he said, "I thought you might have fallen off the face of the earth."

"Some of us have professions, Mr. Logan. And what is this business about a bill?"

"You either shortchanged them or they under-billed me... I mean you, and they came after the rest. No big deal. I've sent the money. How are you?"

"Busy. Busy. Busy. And you?"

"They just took the stitches out today. Doc said it looks great."

She changed the subject. "Are you on the boat? How about dinner tonight?"

"I'm at the Green Parrot and yes." He pulled out his wallet and checked his cash flow by flipping through the Ben Franklins. "Only if you let me buy it, though."

"That's fair enough. You pick."

"That's easy. El Siboney on Catherine Street, not Stock Island. You pick the time."

Then they got disconnected. *Damn*. He tried calling her back. No answer. He had a couple more sips of his drink, then from behind him a sexy voice said, "How about seven?"

Nigel turned. It was Sylvia. "I was just around the corner. What does a girl need to..."

"Trav! Bring the lady the usual."

Travis was quick to pour and handed Sylvia a generous glass of white wine. "Here you go, Ms. Sylvia, our best Pinot Grigio."

"Thank you, Trav. You know what I always say, even the very best isn't good enough." Then she looked at Nigel. "Thank you, darling."

"You're welcome. Are you hungry?"

She leaned in, kissed him on the ear, and whispered, "Starving."

Chapter Ten

Everybody has an opinion; however, Nigel feels El Siboney is Key West's best Cuban restaurant. Hands down. The local Cubans must agree, because they make up most of the patrons.

Nigel ordered vaca frita and water. Sylvia went for another glass of wine and the ropa vieja. They made small talk, mostly about the last couple of weeks. Sylvia did most of the talking since Nigel had little to elaborate on. His daily routine of lying around, taking it easy, and doing a bunch of nothing was boring enough for him. She, on the other hand, went into detail about the messes she had to unravel, from failed rezoning applications and the pulling of incorrect permits to no-shows from contractors and shoddy work from those who did.

"Sometimes I wonder why I even bother anymore," she said.

"Probably because you love it," said Nigel. "I've seen you in action. You feed off the stress, the tension, and the attention you get by being in control."

Sylvia wasn't sure how to take his words and returned a confused look. Nigel picked up on it immediately.

"Don't take that the wrong way. I would imagine that when there are several multi-million-dollar projects going on, and it's your good name on the line, you need to be that way. Yet..."

"Yet what?"

"Yet, much like a light switch, you can turn it off whenever you want. Like when we're alone. You are a different person. In business, you are pushy, savvy, and demanding. In private... you can act quite vulnerable, even needy."

"I am not needy, Nigel Logan."

"I don't mean *needy* as a sign of weakness. I rather like that side of you."

"What are you saying?"

"I'm saying I'm glad I don't have to work with you." He smiled until she returned the same. "I'm afraid my tender ego couldn't take it. I like my Sylvia, not everybody else's."

She reached across the table and took his hand. "Have you ever thought it may be the company I keep that calms me down?"

He squeezed her hand and pulled away as the waiter arrived with their food. With the occasional subtle grunt of satisfaction, they ate in silence until Sylvia caught him staring at her. "What is it?"

Nigel returned an innocent look of guilt.

"What?"

Nigel nodded toward her last uneaten sweet plantain. "You gonna eat that?"

She answered by stabbing it with her fork and popping it into her mouth.

"Damn it."

She laughed as she chewed.

Dinner was excellent as usual, and they ended it by sharing an order of flan and Cuban coffees.

Then a *bong* from Nigel's phone interrupted them. Other people looked at their table. He reached for it with embarrassment. "I meant to put that thing on vibrate."

He looked at the text message. It was from Teddy, the Uber guy.

I'm calling it a night, unless you need me.

Nigel replied. *I think I'm all good here. Enjoy the rest of your evening.*

"That was my driver. He's calling it a night."

"So, I guess that means I'm stuck with you."

Nigel's initial thought was that she could drop him off at the base gate, but on second thought, he recounted the number of wines she had consumed. She wasn't drunk, but she didn't need to be driving either. When they finished their dessert, Nigel reached out his hand and with gentle insistence said, “Keys, please.”

There was no protest.

As he held her car door open, she kissed him on the cheek and climbed in.

Behind the wheel, Nigel said, “I like the new Escalade better than the Jag.”

“I bet you do. It even pained me to see you folded up in that thing. I’d be lying if I said I wasn’t thinking of you when I traded it in.”

“So, you bought it for me?”

“You could say that, and you bought me a tandem bicycle. Where is the equity in that?”

“I’m sorry.”

“Don’t be. Take me home and you can make it up to me.”

Nigel chuckled. “One night? Is my company worth that much?”

“Oh, hell no. You’ll be working this off for a while. Now, take me home.”

And he did.

Chapter Eleven

Nigel woke up under the sheets with Sylvia. She was curled up in a ball by his side. He felt good and refreshed, but needed coffee. The addiction called, so he pulled the sheets back, found Sylvia's noggin, and kissed her forehead. Then he slipped out of bed, found his shorts, and carried them out of the room and downstairs to the kitchen.

She came down the stairs about thirty minutes later and found him sitting on the sofa, nursing a cup. He looked up as she gently descended, rubbing her eyes. "Did I wake you?"

"No. But I was hoping you would."

"I couldn't bring myself to. You were sleeping like an angel."

She cuddled up next to him, pulling her feet beneath her body. "What time is it?"

"About a quarter to five."

"Is there any more of that?" she said, nosing toward his cup.

"Sure."

As he rose and headed to the kitchen, she said, "You let me down last night."

"Is that so? How did I manage that?"

"You were the perfect gentleman."

He poured a cup. "Well, somebody finished a bottle of wine and fell asleep."

"I was exhausted..." she said as she reached up for her cup of coffee. After taking a sip, she continued, "but dammit, I would have felt fine when you woke up. Let's go back to bed."

"Sylvia... Stop it."

"Just my luck to wake up with Eagle Scout Logan."

"Hush. And I never made it past Tenderfoot."

"Speaking of a tender foot."

Nigel lifted his foot in the air and twisted it back and forth. "It's feeling fine. I'm going to try a gentle jog later." He grabbed an inch of his midriff. "I have got to get back into the routine."

"You could come do yoga with me sometime."

He replied with *a look*.

"Anyway, I'm sorry about that pesky bill from Belize."

"It's no big deal. It was a hundred fifty-something bucks. I paid it."

"Well, I'm sorry anyway." She sipped her coffee.

"I wonder how she is doing?"

"Who?"

"Dr. Cabrera. From the clinic in Belize."

"How do you mean?"

Nigel gave her a confused look until the light came on. "Oh, that's right. We haven't talked about her bizarre circumstances. Don't you remember? She was upset. Working on the day *they* buried her husband."

"Yes, come to think of it, but I haven't given it much thought since."

Nigel got up to pace the floor.

"Well, I have. I spoke with her while you were... taking your nap in her office."

He filled in the gaps for her. The strange comment about Venezuela. Her contract with the Henry Reeve Brigade that kept her in Belize, instead of Cuba, where she belonged. How she was even working that day at all.

"It's all so damn weird. I mean, come on. It's one thing to miss your husband's funeral for unforeseen circumstances, but it's another when you're not permitted to attend. I just find it so sad. There is no way to justify it."

"It does sound crazy. What about this brigade stuff?"

"I gave them a Google search and found several articles of praise. Hell, even the World Health Organization gave them an award."

"Humph," grunted Sylvia.

"Exactly. It isn't like we can do anything. I just keep seeing that look she gave me when she felt like she had said too much. She was frightened."

"If it continues to bother you, we could always talk to a friend of mine. He's very connected in the Cuban community. He may shed some light. If anything, maybe he could give us a better understanding."

Nigel was now standing at the big picture window, gazing at the darkness and glow of the streetlights. "Yeah. I think I would like to do that. Where does he live?"

"Miami. He's quite the night owl, so I'll give Basilio a call after lunch."

Nigel nodded his head as he peered out the window. Then something she said made his eyebrows come together. He spun. "Did you say, Basilio?"

"Yeah, Basilio Valdez. Why?"

Nigel turned away so she couldn't see his smile. "Nothing. Odd name. That's all."

Basilio Valdez was a name Nigel wasn't expecting to hear. He figured for a moment that it could be a different Basilio, but brushed that idea to the side as quickly as it came. How many people named Basilio Valdez could there be? Nigel first met Basilio not long after making landfall in Port St. Joe. They were both transient mariners, dockmates at the Port St. Joe Marina, making a temporary stop at the friendly coastal town until they were ready to get underway and move on. Nigel was aboard *MisChief* while Basilio stayed aboard his Grand Banks 42 trawler, *Cubano Freedom*, until it was destroyed. Basilio was in the restaurant and import/export business, and Nigel wondered how much Sylvia knew about the Cuban and his connections and business dealings.

Nigel turned around and went to sit with Sylvia. "So, tell me about your friend, this Basilio?" Nigel studied her face as she spoke.

"He is very involved in matters pertaining to the Cuban community in Miami and elsewhere. He owns several restaurants in Miami and the Keys and is known for his excellent chefs. As a matter of fact, the chef at El Siboney last night... he once worked for Basilio."

"Really? Interesting. You said he was a night owl?"

"And a carouser. Oh my, how the young ladies flock to him, and he loves it."

Nigel smiled, thinking of his first encounter with the Cuban and the fourteen or fifteen coeds from Florida State that were on his boat. "Sounds like my kind of guy."

"Easy, Bucko."

Nigel's mind raced. "So, do you think he will meet with us?"

"With as much money as I've spent entertaining in his restaurants, he better."

Nigel sat thinking and tapping his knee with his fingertips.

"What?" asked Sylvia.

"Do me a favor. When you speak to him, don't mention my name. Just refer to me as a friend. I think that will be best."

"Okay, but why?"

Nigel stood and walked back to look out the window. The eastern sky was just beginning to cast a glow. "Let me ask you a question. Just how much do you know about me?" He watched her reflection in the mirror and watched her head tilt back in thought.

"Enough, I suppose. I'm not going to lie. I had someone look you up and investigate. It was after all the dust settled last year with the Christmas Key issue. Please understand. A single woman in my position can't..."

Nigel turned around. "What? Take any chances? I get it."

"Well, yes. Do you know how many smooth-talking, unscrupulous scoundrels this rock attracts?"

"I can imagine. Listen, I'm not offended, but I am interested in knowing what your investigator reported."

"Cam told me everything. The good. The bad. The ugly. And... the very ugly."

Nigel turned around. "Cam? You had Cam investigate me?"

"Well, yeah! For crying out loud, he's a private investigator. Would you rather it be someone else?"

She made sense. "Probably not."

"That's what I thought."

"So... what was the number one thing you took away from his report?"

"That you are sincere and can be trusted."

"What's the second thing?"

She remained silent for a few beats.

"Well?"

"That you can be dangerous."

Thinking of his old girlfriend, Candice, he said, "I bet I know where he got that idea from."

"Huh?"

"Nothing."

"Nigel, listen... I like you and I think you like me. We have a special, uncomplicated friendship, right?"

"Yeah."

She stood to join him, wrapping her arms around his torso. He did the same and held her tight. "I am a tough and savvy businesswoman," she said. "I am good at what I do, and I don't take crap off anyone."

"I know. You impress me."

"But much of what people see is an act. A front to look strong."

"I know that too. You can't fool me."

She pulled away to look at him. "I feel safe when I'm with you."

"Understood. I'm glad I make you feel secure. So... with that, we don't know what may become of our meeting with your friend. What did you say his name was again?"

"Basilio. I understand he can be dangerous, too."

"Yes, so maybe you will understand why I might not want him to know my name just yet."

"What if he insists?"

"If he must know, tell him my name is Jim Horton. It's a popular alias I sometimes use."

"Okay. Will do. It's still hours before I can call him. Will you join me in the shower before I have to get ready for work?"

He reached down and picked her up. "Hold tight."

Chapter Twelve

Nigel sat in the salon of *MisChief*. A bottle of fifteen-year-old Havana Club sat on the table. It was authentic, not the stuff made by Bacardi and sold in the United States. No, it was the real deal and what remained from a case he acquired from his old Cuban friend just before he disappeared years before. The Cuban instructed Nigel to save one bottle for them to share in the future. He had been toting that bottle around for years, never knowing if he would ever get to crack the seal. There was a time, not so long ago, when Nigel's appetite for alcohol was greater than his inventory. He often eyed that last bottle, but for some reason, he would push back his temptation back where it belonged. Not out of willpower, though. He always found another solution nearby.

He shook his head, trying to do the math. *If it was fifteen when bottled, hell, how old is it now?* He looked at the overhead in thought. *Crap, I do not know. Over twenty, for sure.* His phone interrupted his thoughts. It rang, and it was Sylvia.

"We're on for dinner tonight," she said.

"Where?"

"The Real Habana on Lower Matecumbe Key at seven. He said he was extremely busy and probably couldn't meet until next week. Then I gave him a little background, and his interest piqued. Once I mentioned the Henry Reeve organization, holy shit, that changed everything and he can't wait to meet us, Mr. Horton."

Nigel smiled. "Perfect."

"Pick you up at the gate at five."

As he saw the new Escalade come around the bend, Nigel stood and shouldered a backpack. He had been leaning up against one of the large concrete security barriers positioned in front of the main gate.

"Is that your ride, Chief?" asked the gate guard.

Nigel turned. "Yeah. Beats that damn Uber. Huh?"

"I'd say so."

The Caddy stopped and Sylvia got out, left the driver's side door open, walked around, and got in the passenger side.

"I guess you're driving, Chief."

Nigel started walking. "Seems to be the case. Keep an eye on my bike. I should be back in a few hours."

"Aye. Aye."

Nigel climbed in. His seat was warm, as was the steering wheel. "Wow," he said. "My old Bronco doesn't have heated anything. Hell, it barely heats the cabin. Luckily, the need in Florida isn't critical."

"But it feels good, doesn't it?"

"Yeah, initially, but I'd rather not meet with your friend with sweaty balls, so do me a favor, will you?"

He put the SUV in drive, and she pushed some buttons on the console, uttering, "Oh my God," under her breath.

They got there about fifteen minutes early, and the sound of the broken oyster shell parking lot sounded especially loud. Maybe because the parking lot was completely empty.

"Is the place even open?" asked Nigel.

"I know it does breakfast and lunch," she said. "I figured he expanded their hours or something."

Moments later Nigel saw a large, bigger-than-life figure emerge from the front door and porch, waving them in. It was Basilio. The Cuban. Nigel grabbed the bill of his cap and pulled it down to hide his eyes. Then they got out.

As he and Sylvia approached, Basilio said, "Ms. Sylvia! You look as beautiful as ever. Welcome!"

Climbing the porch steps, Sylvia said, "And you are kind with your flattery, as usual."

"Please. Please. Come in. I'm having Javier fix us something special." He turned, headed inside, and held open the door.

Once inside, it was time for introductions. Nigel tried to keep his head down without making it obvious. "Basilio," she started, "this is my friend..." She hesitated slightly, trying to remember the name. "Jim, Jim Horton. Jim, this is the man I spoke of... my friend Basilio Valdez."

Basilio stretched out a hand, and with that old, familiar, booming voice said, "Pleasure to meet you, sir."

Nigel took Basilio's hand and slowly raised his head until their eyes met. Nigel's face was cheerful. Basilio's was confused and searching. With his free hand, Basilio lifted the bill of Nigel's hat to see better. Nigel let him. Then Nigel felt the Cuban's grip tighten as his laughter filled the room. The next thing Nigel knew, Basilio pulled him into a massive bear hug.

"My friend! My friend! It has been too long."

Sylvia said, "What? What is going on?"

Nigel and Basilio ignored her.

Nigel tried to return the hug but couldn't since he was having a hard time catching his breath. He coughed out, "Bas... ili... o. Goo... d to... see you... too?"

Basilio freed his embrace. "Let me look at you," he said. "My, you haven't changed a bit."

Sylvia's fists were now squarely on her hips. "Would someone please tell me what in the hell is going on?"

Basilio released Nigel and took Sylvia into his arms. "His name is not Horton." A look of concern stretched across his face. "Has he been lying to you?" But in an instant, the smile was back. "This is my dear old friend, Nigel Logan."

"Dear old friend?" said Sylvia. "You two know each other?" She looked at Nigel. "How can that be?"

"Long story," said Nigel.

"I feel like a fool."

Nigel pulled her into a hug. "Don't. You couldn't have known. I'll tell you all about it later. I promise." He kissed her on the forehead. When he turned around, Basilio had his arms crossed.

"Mr. Logan, we have some business to discuss."

"That we do, but not without a drink."

Nigel picked up the backpack that had found its way to the floor during the hugfest. He opened the zipper and produced the bottle of Havana Club. "I was beginning to wonder if I'd ever get to open this."

Basilio slowly approached with a grin and took the bottle. "You did as I asked. You saved us a bottle."

Nigel nodded.

"After all this time, that had to be a difficult thing to do."

"You don't know."

"You two know each other." Sylvia was still shaking her head. "I can't believe this. Logan... you're an asshole. Jim Horton... what a heap of bullshit."

"I'm sorry, Sylvia," said Nigel. "I promise to make it up to you."

"That hole of debt just gets deeper and deeper. You haven't even made the first payment on the Escalade!"

"I know not what you two speak of," said Basilio with scrunched eyebrows, "but I can tell you this much Ms. Sylvia..." He grabbed Nigel around the waist and pulled him close to his side, "this is a good and sincere man. And I am thrilled to see him."

"See," said Nigel. "Just like Cam said."

With the other hand, Basilio raised the bottle of old rum in the air. "More importantly, he keeps his promises and is loyal to his friends."

"Oh, he's a regular choir boy for sure," said Sylvia. "What about being dangerous?"

Basilio cut his curious eyes at Nigel.

"Yeah," said Nigel, "she knows."

Basilio returned his gaze to Sylvia. "The only thing I will say about that is, he does that very well, too."

Releasing Nigel, Basilio said, "As much as I would love to know how you two met, and as much as Sylvia would like to know our history, Nigel, we can catch up on that later. We agreed to meet to discuss more serious matters, if I recall. Follow me to the back deck and you can fill me in."

As they walked through the restaurant, Basilio barked. "Javier! Two glasses, a bucket of ice, and a long pour of Pinot Grigio, please. We'll be out on the veranda."

Chapter Thirteen

Sylvia excused herself to visit the powder room as they crossed through the dining room. As the two sat, Javier emerged to deliver the goods. Basilio gave a nod and Javier dashed back to the kitchen. "He is an excellent chef and preparing his favorite roasted pork dish for us tonight. I am sure you will find it to be the best to ever cross your palate."

"I expect nothing less. So... how long have you had this one?"

"I grabbed him last year. He is so appreciative to be in America and free of the oppression."

"I'm sure. So, before she gets back, how much does Sylvia know about your little import/export endeavors?"

"Thank you for asking. She knows nothing, and it should remain that way."

Nigel nodded, "As you wish."

Basilio lowered his head to extend his appreciation.

"Basilio, the last time we saw each other, you were going into hiding. How long were you away?"

"Ahh, about eighteen months. The regime and I now have an accord. If they keep their operatives and assassins out of my business, I will continue to let them live."

"They agreed to that?"

"No, but they know keenly that I am serious. But in a show of good faith, I haven't exported another chef since Javier."

"Well, I guess they appreciate that. So, you're giving up the chef smuggling business?"

"Export Nigel. Export. How many times do I have to tell you?"

Nigel stood. "Here she comes."

Basilio rose too, and he handed her the glass of wine. "Please, everyone, remain standing." Basilio grabbed the rum, broke the seal, removed the cork, and poured a generous amount for both him and Nigel. He picked up his glass. "We toast."

Nigel looked down at his rum, hesitated, then picked it up.

"To old friends and new adventures," said Basilio.

They clinked their glasses and took a sip. "Please... sit."

Nigel stepped around to assist Sylvia with her chair, then the men sat and joined her.

"Nigel, Sylvia has provided me with a little background, but she feels you could explain things in clearer detail. As I understand it, you were fortunate enough to receive some special emergency care from some of our finest healthcare workers."

"Yes. The care was excellent. I'm not sure what Sylvia told you, so let me start from the beginning."

He explained everything to Basilio, including the details that Dr. Cabrera had provided until the point where she felt she had said too much. As he spoke, Nigel could see aggravation building on Basilio's face. Nigel shared details that were stoking a fire.

"It was all so strange, Basilio. They did not allow her to return to Cuba for her husband's funeral. I mean, what is that all about? And her comments about her husband staying in Venezuela. Did his leaving get him killed? I spent a little time looking up this Henry Reeve Medical Brigade. There is no shortage of online accolades. They seem highly regarded around..."

And that was when Basilio lost it. His fist came crashing down on the table. Nigel and Sylvia gave a jump. Rum sloshed out of their glasses and Sylvia's wine fell over and spilled. The white tablecloth absorbed everything.

"Bullshit! It is all bullshit!" Basilio stood and paced the deck with his arms crossed. Nigel and Sylvia let him. After three or four trips back and forth, he stopped at the table. "I'll tell you what it is... government-sponsored slavery. Blatant slavery for everyone to see."

"What?" asked Nigel.

"Nigel. Listen to me. It is a state-sponsored labor pool. The communist Cuban government forces many of their talented medical professionals and others into contracts with other countries. Many countries are oblivious to the terms, other more corrupt states couldn't care less. The brigade often shows up to provide much-needed care in cases of natural disasters, like hurricanes and mudslides. In fact, the brigade was formed in 2005 on the heels of Hurricane Katrina. Fidel offered their services to President Bush in response to the disaster, but he would have nothing to do with it and gently gave Castro the middle finger. Since then, the brigade has continued to do its great work. As a devout Cuban, I am very proud of my people, but it all comes at a price. Don't believe all the propaganda, my friend. The bastards are profiting off the talents of my people."

"Why don't they just flee once outside of Cuba?" asked Sylvia.

"Coercion, my dear. Once in the country, they are restricted and held in a controlled environment. The regime confiscates their passports and withholds seventy-five to ninety percent of their pay until the mission is complete and they return to Cuba."

Nigel looked confused.

"Yes. You heard me correctly. The host country is not responsible for their pay. The doctors are provided with room and board and a small stipend from their normal pay for incidentals. It is criminal."

"And the Cuban government profits?" asked Nigel.

Basilio lowered his head and drifted it from side to side. Then he looked up. "The host countries pay the regime a monthly fee per medical professional. Anywhere from three thousand to fourteen thousand dollars."

"Fourteen thousand a month!" exclaimed Sylvia.

"I'll put it this way, my sweet friend. Doctors and nurses have become my country's most lucrative export. To the tune of almost eleven billion dollars annually."

"That is incredible," said Nigel.

"Why isn't there more public outcry?" asked Sylvia.

"The propaganda. Nigel has seen it. There is no shortage of news articles touting the altruistic work provided by the brigade. And while the efforts of my people might be altruistic, the same cannot be said for the regime. Bastards."

"And they just can't leave? Run away?"

"Where would they go? They have no passport for travel, and they have no money to sustain themselves. Plus, if they run and leave their post, the regime considers them deserters, and forbidden to return to Cuba for eight years. If they do return, they face harsh punishment."

Sylvia and Nigel said nothing.

"My friends... my people... your Dr. Cabrera, and many others are trapped. Trapped with no good way to get out except to complete their assigned missions and return to Cuba."

Nigel and Sylvia exchanged glances.

Basilio looked down at the table, and at some point, unbeknownst to anyone, Javier slipped in and delivered their meals. "Oh my, please eat. I hope it hasn't gotten cold. But before we do..." He raised his glass of rum. Nigel and Sylvia did the same. "To my people. God, bless them and keep them safe."

The food was exceptional, but their appetites had waned. All three ate in silence, taking small bites from time to time. It was a shame to waste such an excellent meal, but the gravity of the conversation diminished their hunger and enjoyment.

Finally, Sylvia asked, "What can be done?"

Basilio cut Nigel a curious look, and Nigel sent a silent message with his eyes. *No.*

Basilio returned his focus to Sylvia. "I'm afraid there isn't much *we* can do." Which was the truth. *They* couldn't do anything. Basilio, on the other hand... Well, that was another story.

"I'm sorry," said Nigel. "I wasn't sure what to expect from our little reunion, but I certainly didn't mean to come and upset you."

Basilio stood, stepped away from the table, and held his arms out. Returning to his normal, jovial demeanor, said, "Come here my friend."

Nigel got up, joined his old comrade, and fell into his embrace. "Not too tight," he begged.

But Basilio would have none of it. He squeezed and lifted Nigel's frame off the floor. Most of the vertebrae in Nigel's back popped. "It has been so good to see you, my friend. What a pleasant surprise."

Nigel hissed, "Good to see you too."

The Cuban released Nigel and turned to Sylvia. "You are as beautiful as ever, and thank you for bringing Nigel to me. It made my day, and I apologize to you both for ruining our dinner. Oh, how I get carried away sometimes. I'll see you to the door."

As they walked out on the front patio, Nigel used the key fob to unlock the Caddy. Sylvia descended the stairs.

Basilio grabbed Nigel's hand and pulled him into another friendly embrace.

Nigel felt Basilio slip something into his hand. And as they were close, Basilio whispered. "Call me tomorrow."

Basilio released his friend, and Nigel looked down at the card in his palm. Nigel nodded.

Chapter Fourteen

Nigel crawled out of the v-berth the next morning feeling exhausted. Sleep hadn't come easy. Basilio's words ran through his brain like a gerbil on a steel-caged treadmill in dire need of oiling. He lit up his wristwatch: 0342. It was almost time to get up anyway. After starting some coffee, he removed the hatch boards and proceeded to the end of the dock. The marina was quiet and still. Most places are at that time of the morning. The other places, the ones that never sleep or slow down, must be a glimpse into hell.

The water was like a dark mirror reflecting the star canopy above. Scattered lamp posts throughout the marina cast a dim glow down on the docks. Somewhere in the distance, a rooster was starting his day, too. Wearing only a t-shirt, Nigel closed his eyes and filled his lungs, taking in the smells of the low tide. Then he watered the ducks.

The gurgle of the coffee pot told him the morning nectar was almost ready, so he prepared his favorite cup with a generous pour of heavy cream. As the pot coughed one last time, he pulled the pot and poured. The envelope on the counter caught his eye. He picked it up on the way into the salon.

That first sip of fresh, hot coffee is the best. Nigel made it count. Then he turned his attention to the envelope. In it was the card and picture from Red. He looked at the image of his friend amongst the pile of fish. It made him laugh. "I miss you too, brother," he said to the picture.

He missed all his St. Joe family, even that annoying, beer-drinking, television-watching, four-legged Weedeater of a goat named Maxine. Nigel thought about the date and time. *Has it really been over a year since I left?* He looked at the picture again. Then grabbed his phone. As he scrolled through his contact list, he looked at his watch: 0417. Nigel smiled and hit the phone icon to dial.

The phone on the other end rang several times before going to voicemail. He ended the call without leaving a message and hit dial again. Three rings into the transmission, a groggy and aggravated voice on the other end said, "If your ass needs bailing out, call Trixie, dammit."

The abrupt dead silence that followed told Nigel that his buddy had ended the call.

Nigel chuckled and called again.

Trixie is Red's wife. She owns and operates Trixie's Freedom Bail Bonds, a popular local service. Not only for the attentive customer service, but for the complimentary, international orange t-shirt that says... *I Got My Freedom at Trixie's!* Everybody could use a free t-shirt.

Red, on the other hand, is the owner and headmaster of a private facility of higher education: R.I.D.D. Red's Institute for Drunk Drivers.

When Red picked up, Nigel spoke first. "Don't hang up. I can't sleep. There's something I have to say."

Red raised his head and let his eyes adjust to the darkness to read. The red digital numbers on the alarm clock made his head flop down on his pillow. "You can't sleep because you're finished sleeping. I'm not."

"I know. I know," said Nigel. "But this can't wait. I must get this off my chest. It's about the nice card and picture you sent me."

"Really? Can't it wait till morning?"

"It is morning, Red."

Red closed his eyes, took a deep breath, and exhaled, saying, "What is it, then?"

"It's the picture, Red. It's bullshit. You've never netted that much mullet in your life. Or at least as long as I've known you."

Red's eyes popped back open. "That's it? That's what you found so important that you had to call and wake me up?"

From the other side of the bed, Nigel heard the husky voice of Trixie utter, "That includes me. Thanks for nothing."

Red tilted his head. "It's Nigel, Trix."

Trixie sat up on her elbows and grunted, "Nigel? ... Is everything alright?"

"Apparently."

Nigel heard their little conversation. "Good morning, Trixie!"

Red looked at her. "He said..."

"I heard him." Then she raised her voice a notch. "Good morning to you too, hon."

"Trix, aren't you just a little pissed that he called to wake us up for nothing?"

"Oh, shut up, Red."

"What can I say, Red?" said Nigel. "Being a favorite comes with certain privileges."

Red huffed.

"Besides," said Nigel. "Your phony baloney picture isn't the main reason I called..."

"It wasn't a phony!"

"Whatever. You'll have to prove me wrong sometime, but the main reason I called is to say... I miss you and Trixie too. There I said it. You can go back to sleep now."

Trixie snatched the phone from Red and put it on speaker. "When are you coming home?"

"I don't know."

"But how are you doing?"

"I'm doing fine. I think Key West has been good for me. If you can believe that."

Trixie said nothing.

"How is..." Nigel stammered, "um... Candice? How is she?"

Candice was Nigel's longtime girlfriend in St. Joe. It took her time to win him over, but she finally did. And he fell all in, even when he knew better.

His secret life and past hung over him like a shroud of darkness, and as time moved on, there was no hiding who he was and the violence he was capable of. In the end, she could no longer handle her fears that were created by the dangers that constantly pulled at him. It wasn't that she didn't love him. It was that she couldn't let herself love him anymore, so she pushed him away.

Her timing couldn't have been worse. He was already having a difficult time coming to terms with who he had become. Not a killer, just somebody capable and willing if the circumstances warranted it. He didn't ask for that life, but he took ownership of it. And what tormented him the most was how comfortable he felt in that role. He couldn't blame Candice for ending it, but it stung his heart. To cope, he turned down a disastrous road; an increase in his already abusive consumption of beer and booze. To save himself, he needed to get away. Setting sail from Port St. Joe was a must.

"She is doing fine. She misses you, though she would never admit it."

"Well, the next time you see her, let her know I asked. Not that I think she would care."

"Come home, Nigel," said Trixie. "This is where you belong."

"You might be right, but not yet. Trixie... I'm just not ready to come back. Besides, the Keys will never be home, but this place is growing on me."

"You met somebody!"

Her words reached Nigel as a statement more than a question, so he said nothing.

"What's her name?"

"Sylvia, and we are just good friends."

"Sylvia what?"

There was no way he would reveal Sylvia's last name. He knew Trixie all too well. She would have Sylvia researched and fully vetted before the end of her morning coffee, so he dodged the question. "We met last year, before Christmas." He smiled. "She and Santa got into a little trouble and a friend, and I had to rally the elves."

"You're so full of crap, Nigel Logan."

"I know. I know. Some things never change. Listen, I better go so y'all can get back to sleep."

"Go back to sleep?" said Red. "How in the hell are we supposed to do that?"

Trixie gave Red a little backhanded swat. "Stop being such a grumpy ass, Red."

Nigel laughed.

"Listen to Trixie. Come home and we'll throw the nets."

Bong! It was a text. Nigel looked at the name: *Basilio*.

"I'd love to, Red. Soon maybe, but right now I have a feeling I may be a little busy around here."

Trixie gave a huff. "A little busy, huh? Why is it I don't like the sounds of that?"

"It's nothing like that," said Nigel, hoping he was lying. "That's all for now. Love you guys. Got to run."

"We love you too," said Trixie. "Be safe."

"Ahh, hell, that takes all the fun out of it."

"And that's what worries us," said Red.

"Goodbye now and stop your fussing." Nigel ended the call.

Chapter Fifteen

Basilio answered before Nigel ever heard the first ring. “I don’t like it, my friend. I don’t like it at all.”

“What did you find out?”

“They killed him.”

“Dr. Cabrera’s husband?”

“Exactly.”

“Who would have done something like that?”

“If I had to guess, the ministry or someone within the ministry. His name was Alejandro. He too had been a doctor in the brigade.”

“But he was in Venezuela?”

“Yes. He and another man were found dead in Palmira, Cuba. A town outside the city of Cienfuegos.”

“What ministry?”

“MININT… The Ministry of Interior. They maintain control and order over domestic unrest and pretty much everything else. Bastards. All of them. Some, more than others.”

“Why would they kill him?”

“Details are still coming in. I have people on the ground looking into it. But remember, the good doctor in Belize said her husband should have stayed in Venezuela, so obviously she was right.”

“What now?”

“Until I know more, there isn’t much to do. But…”

"But what?" asked Nigel, squinting with one eye and raising the eyebrow of the other.

"I was thinking you might want to go back to Belize. She wanted you to keep a follow-up appointment, no?"

"Yeah… here in the States."

Basilio said nothing.

Nigel could hear him breathing, so he knew he was still there. The quiet was more than Nigel could stand. "And you can't go because…"

"Because it wouldn't be smart. Basilio Valdez is far too known to the MININT agents."

"Well shit, Basilio! What do you have in mind?"

"We need to get her a message and monitor her circumstances. How does she come and go? Who is watching her? I know, especially now, they will watch her more closely than before. Probably by MININT agents from the embassy."

Now it was Nigel's turn to say nothing.

"Will you help me?"

"You know Basilio, I sort of made a promise to myself and an old girlfriend once that I was going to get out of this kind of business."

"And what kind of business are you referring to?"

"The business of trouble, Basilio. I tend to embrace it."

"Nigel, all I am asking you is to check on her, make sure she is safe, and deliver a message."

"What would you like for her to know?"

"Basically, that she is not alone, there is hope, and that her countrymen are looking out for her. Once I know more of what we are up against, I'm sure there will be more."

"You keep saying, *we*."

"I can't do this alone, Nigel."

"I know. That's what scares me."

"Ha! Nigel Logan scared? That, my friend, is funny."

"There have been plenty of times when I had no reason to laugh."

"So, will you help me?"

"Call me when you know more."

Chapter Sixteen

When the second pot of coffee finished brewing, Nigel looked at his watch. 0615. Only two hours into his new day, and already so much had happened. He poured another cup and went outside to sit in *MisChief's* cockpit. The sun would rise soon, and he wanted to be there. Not that he could see it from his slip, but he enjoyed watching the daylight develop.

As he sat there drinking his beans, two comments bounced around in his head: Basilio asking if he would help, and Trixie telling him to come home. He deeply wanted the latter, but wasn't sure he was ready. Hell, he wasn't even sure what *being ready* would look like, and not *being ready* bothered him. He always felt ready for anything, no matter what.

"Screw it," he said aloud. "Maybe I should just tell Basilio, 'Thanks, but no thanks!' I'll settle with the harbormaster. Then, set sail for St. Joe." Suddenly, that sounded like a great idea. Yes, it did. The more it soaked into his gray matter, the more excited he got. He knocked down the rest of the coffee and went below for another cup. He paused and looked to the east. The sky had brightened. So had his spirits. He smiled.

As he poured another cup with his free hand, he grabbed his cell phone. Red answered after four rings.

"Son of a bitch! What does a guy have to do to get some rest around here?"

"I thought you said you couldn't go back to sleep."

"Well, give me credit for trying. What now?"

"Where is Trix?"

Red looked around the room, then heard the shower. "She's in the bathroom getting ready for work."

"Shouldn't you be doing the same?"

"My first class of drunks isn't until the afternoon. Two o'clock. What do you need?"

"Just tell Trixie to call me before she heads to the office." Then Nigel ended the call without saying goodbye. He was that excited. Then a sobering thought crossed his mind. *Sylvia*. They both knew that they were a temporary item, but Nigel never figured his decision to return home would be so spontaneous. He sent her a text. *Dinner tonight?*

He grabbed a fistful of hair and laughed. There was so much to do. He had to get provisions for the trip, top off with fresh water and diesel. Diving to clean and inspect *MisChief's* bottom would be a good idea, too.

Bong!

He grabbed his phone and looked at the text. It was from Sylvia. *Where and what time?*

He used his thumbs to type. *I'm flexible. You pick. Anywhere you would like and dinner is on me.*

Bong!

Wow. My choice? Are we celebrating something?

You could say that. Just say where and when.

Bong!

Blue Heaven six thirty.

Then the phone started ringing, and he typed fast. *Se yu hen.*

"Trixie! Thanks for calling back."

"That's fine. What do you need?"

Red kept his head down on his pillow but looked at Trixie with one eye open. He watched her listen to Nigel and saw a tear fall from her eyes. Her lips quivered, and she pressed them with her free fingers.

"What is it?" asked Red, now sitting up on an elbow.

Trixie waved at Red and mouthed, *Hush*.

"Are you sure, Nigel?" She listened some more.

"That is wonderful. I understand, and thank you for calling." She ended the call.

"What is it, dammit?" Red demanded.

Trixie turned and looked at Red. "He said for you to get the nets ready. He's coming home."

"Coming home, but he said..."

"I know what he said earlier, Red."

"When?"

She covered her mouth. "As soon as possible. He said he would set sail tomorrow if the weather cooperated."

"I wonder what made him change his mind."

"Don't know. Don't care. All I know is your buddy is coming home. I can't wait to tell everybody."

"Telling everybody? Huh! Trix, that's your favorite pastime."

WHACK!

Chapter Seventeen

Teddy, Nigel's Uber guy, pulled up to the front gate where Nigel waited. Nigel opened the door and flopped in the front seat.

"Tired of riding the bike into town?" asked Teddy.

"No. Not sure I'll need it or you later for the trip back."

"Oh. Another hot date with Ms. Mason, huh?"

"Mind your own business."

"You are my business, Chief. Where to?"

"Blue Heaven."

Nigel chuckled as Teddy shifted into drive.

He was quieter than normal on the ride into town. Teddy picked up on this and joined him. Nigel gazed out the window and over the water as they crossed the bridge to Stock Island. He thought of his time in Key West. It had been good for him. Despite all the temptations, he had mostly remained sober, only having a sip here and there and maybe an infrequent glass of red wine that he would nurse throughout an entire evening. Yes, indeed, his previous imaginary desires and physiological need for booze had waned.

He was strong, fit, and of good mind. There was something else, too. Something still new and quite foreign, a heightened level of spirituality. It had hit him when he was at his lowest, over a year ago, back in St. Joe. It solidified later when he and Cam chased down an unimaginable kidnapper who had taken Sylvia and Santa hostage. *Old Sinter.* He missed that old man.

Nigel laughed out loud, thinking of him.

"You okay, Chief?" asked Teddy.

Nigel looked at him. "Yeah! I'm fine. Let me ask you something."

"Shoot."

"Do you believe in Santa Claus?"

Teddy answered with a tilt of the head and raised eyebrows.

Nigel looked back out the window and said, "Well, you should."

Teddy said nothing.

"Hey, buddy, when we roll onto the island, take South Roosevelt. I want to ride by the water."

"You got it."

Moments later, Teddy turned left.

Nigel smiled as he gazed out over the water toward the Florida Straits and, ultimately, Cuba. Thoughts of Havana made him think of Belize and Dr. Cabrera. A quick chill of sadness ran through his veins, but two thoughts brought the warmth back. Knowing Basilio would make things right and that he himself would soon sail the same waters back to St. Joe. As the car made the bend onto Bertha Street, Nigel sat up straighter, looked forward, and said, "Thanks, Teddy."

After weaving through the streets of Key West, Teddy stopped at the corner curb of Petronia and Thomas. "Here we are!" he announced.

Nigel looked out the window toward the restaurant, then toward Teddy. From his pocket, Nigel pulled out a hundred-dollar bill and offered it to his driver.

Teddy looked at the cash. "What is this?"

"It's yours, Teddy. It has been a pleasure having you drive Ms. Daisy around town for the past several months. This may be the last time I need your services, and I just wanted to thank you properly."

Teddy kept staring at the Franklin.

Nigel poked it at him. "Take it! Before I shove it up your ass."

He did. "I don't understand."

"I'm leaving the Keys, Teddy. I'm going home. If it holds, tomorrow's forecast is perfect. I'll have a nice brisk northeasterly that will carry *Mis-Chief* and me out of town."

"Mischief?"

"My boat. I live on a sailboat. Have I not shared that with you?"

Teddy shook his head.

"Well, I do, and we're pulling out in the morning." Nigel reached out, and they shook hands.

"It's been my pleasure, Chief."

"Likewise." Nigel got out and before closing the door said, "If I should need you later, you'll know tonight didn't go quite as planned."

"You got this, Chief."

Nigel chuckled as he watched Teddy ride off. Then he turned and walked in the main entrance. It led to the patio where folks can eat and listen to live music coming off the stage. Nigel smiled as he approached the hostess. Her dark tan and blond hair with blue highlights made him think of his old girlfriend, Candice. He knew she would have approved of the hostess's selection of color. He read her name tag. "Hello, Margo. The name is Logan. I have a five thirty reservation." He looked at his watch. "I know I'm a little early, but..." He watched as Margo smiled and shook her head. "What?"

Margo used her thumb to point over her shoulder. "She beat you to it."

Nigel looked around and found Sylvia standing at a table with a glass of wine. He gave a little huff, then looked at Margo. "Thank you, sweetheart." Nigel walked on past and, after a few steps, stopped and turned around. "And Margo..."

She turned to face him.

"I like your hair. It reminds me of a friend."

She blushed, pulled at a section of blue, and said, "Gee. Thanks."

He gave her a wink, then joined Sylvia by giving her a kiss on the cheek.

"You're early," she said.

"You're earlier."

Nigel helped with her chair as she sat. Nigel took the chair across from her.

"So," she said, "we are celebrating?"

"Yeah, you could say that. At least I am."

"Do tell."

Nigel sat in quiet reflection for a moment before speaking. He took in her curious but happy expression. "Well, before I start, let me say I think you are an amazing woman. And personally, I feel fortunate to have been pulled into your company. The past year or so, especially since Christmas…"

"Uh-oh. What is going on?"

"I'm ready to… go sailing…"

"Duh!"

"… back to St. Joe."

"Oh! St. Joe. You mean you are leaving?"

Nigel slowly nodded his head with a slight tilt. "Yeah. I miss my people and my old way of life."

"But you have a way of life here."

"I do. And it's been wonderful. It just isn't the same. I'm ready for… familiarity."

"Wow. I wasn't expecting this."

"Me either, not until early this morning. I realized over coffee. I need to get back."

"I'm sad and disappointed, but not mad. I understand… I think." She smiled and reached across the table for his hand, and he gave it to her.

A waitress approached. "May I get the gentleman something to drink?"

"Nigel," said Sylvia, "this is our server, Lily. She is just the sweetest thing."

Nigel nodded. "My pleasure, Lily. And I'd like a Diet Coke, please. Dress it up with a lime."

Lily smiled and rolled her eyes. "Fancy."

"He's an exotic and wild one, Lil. Be careful."

Lily turned to get his drink and Sylvia said, "So, what happens if you get back to St. Joe and this familiarity you seek isn't there? It's just a question. Asking for a friend."

"I don't think I have to worry about that. The place hasn't changed a bit. There's a reason it is called The Forgotten Coast. I mean, the entire county only has three traffic lights. Two of them are in St. Joe."

"The town might not have changed, but what about you?"

She was right, and he knew it. He had changed, for the better he hoped, but he couldn't be sure. "You're right. I'm not the same guy I was over a year ago, and that could make my going home something unexpected and different. But I need to see for myself."

"Of course you do. So, what will you do?"

"What? If it isn't the same?"

"That was sort of the original question."

Nigel got quiet to contemplate. "I don't know," he said. "We'll just have to see, but I don't want to think about it. I prefer to stay positive."

"As you should."

They had a lovely time and a wonderful meal. They shared the Caribbean "BBQ" shrimp as an appetizer and later dug into their entrees. She ordered the filet, and he had the yellow snapper. Both were excellent. They enjoyed many laughs as they shared the many memories they had created over the past few months.

As things wound down, she said, "Thank you for such a wonderful evening. I must admit that I wasn't expecting to say goodbye. You caught me off guard on that one, Nigel Logan."

Nigel heard it in her voice. There would be no last night together. He could accept that. As much as he wanted to hold her one last time, it was probably for the best, anyway. At least she wasn't mad.

"You'll stay *my friend*, right?" he asked.

She stood, and he almost fell over, getting to his feet. He stood his ground as she walked around the table to join him. As she drew near, he opened his arms, and she fell into his embrace. At least he would get to hold her one last time.

"I'm going to miss you, dammit," she said. "It's been a long time since I have felt like this, so be proud of yourself, Mr. Logan."

He held her tight and said, "Kiss me."

She shook her head. "No. This is how I want it to end. Just hug me for now."

He did, and the tighter he squeezed, the harder she squeezed back. As he felt her embrace lessen, he eased his hold on her until they were looking at each other.

"Goodbye, Nigel Logan. You will call from time to time, right?"

"Of course. You're my newest best friend."

She laughed. "Yes. The best of friends." She took his hands into hers, gave them a little shake, bent down, and kissed his fingers. "So long, Chief."

A lump formed in Nigel's throat as he watched her turn and walk away. It was a good walk, and he was sure she was doing it on purpose. *Dammit.*

Lily showed up. "Is everything alright?"

"Everything is fine. Thanks. I'll take the ticket now."

"There is no ticket, Mr. Logan."

"What do you mean?"

Lily said nothing.

"I know Lil, stupid question." *Shit. She did it to me again.*

"I wasn't expecting to hear from you tonight," said Teddy. "Things didn't go as planned, huh?"

"No, but everything is alright. How far out are you?"

"It'll be a few minutes. I have a rider going to Geiger Key Marina."

"That's fine. There is a bench out front facing Thomas Street. I'll cop-a-squat and wait. No hurry."

Several minutes passed by while Nigel reflected on the evening and his time in Key West. This town had grown on him. There was no doubt about that. He couldn't be sure of when, but he knew he would return some day. It may only be for a few days or a week, or maybe another year. Who knows?

Bong!

Nigel smiled at the name on the screen.

Where are you?

Right where you left me.

Bong!

Don't you dare move a damn muscle.

Minutes later, the black Escalade came roaring down Petronia Street, broke hard, and turned toward Thomas. Nigel stood. Then the big SUV came to a screeching halt in the middle of the intersection, blocking traffic. The driver's side door opened and Sylvia got out. She ran around the front of the vehicle and made a beeline for Nigel. The closer she got, the more he could tell she had been crying hard. Her eyes were swollen and most of her mascara streaked down her cheeks. She was still sobbing uncontrollably when she stopped in front of him. Cars stuck at the intersection blew their horns. She didn't care. They could wait.

When she caught her breath, she said, "You are a sorry son of a bitch. Did you know that?"

"I've been called worse."

She threw the car keys high in the air and turned around to head back to the car. When she heard Nigel catch the keys, she barked, "You're driving, dammit!"

He smiled and sent Teddy a quick text.

Chapter Eighteen

At 1007, the Naval Air Station Key West gate guard, Airman Charlie Williams, watched the black Escalade pull up and stop by the gate. He saw the driver and passenger side doors open, with Chief Logan and a beautiful woman getting out to switch sides. At least the woman, anyway.

They met out in front of the grill and immediately went into a hug.

"I am so going to miss you," she said. "And not just for the..." She winked and bit her bottom lip.

Nigel gave a huff. "You are something else, you know that?"

"No. I mean it. I will miss your company more than anything."

"And I will miss you, too. Who knows, maybe if we hadn't vowed to maintain our independence, not get too overly involved, this leaving might be impossible."

She got all sassy, stepped back, and spread her arms out. "Hey, mister. It would take one hell of a man to tie all this down. I've only ever met two men in my entire life. One was my ex-husband, and he's in prison. Good riddance." She moved back in for another hug and placed her head against his chest. "The other, I'm afraid to say, is walking out of my life."

He kissed her on the top of the head. "I'm not walking out of your life. I'm walking back into mine."

"Please tell me you will come back and visit."

Nigel said, "I promise."

"Then kiss me and get the hell out of here. You're a bore."

Nigel reached down and held her face and kissed her one last time. She reached around with both hands and grabbed his butt, giving him a little goose. He backed away from the kiss and noticed the gate guard. "Hey, cut that out. The kids are watching."

Sylvia looked at the gate guard and gave him a wink.

Embarrassed for getting caught, the young airman looked at his feet and kicked at the ground.

Nigel gave her one last kiss and slapped her on the ass. "Go on now. Get."

She walked around, got in the SUV, and rolled down the window. "Promise me you will call to let me know you made it."

"I will. And hey! It's a two-way street, you know. You could come and visit me. We'll run the beaches in my Bronco, and I'll show you how to throw a cast net."

"Sounds dreadful."

"Don't knock it..."

"Goodbye Nigel Logan."

"Goodbye Sylvia Mason."

She backed away and drove off, letting the floodgate of tears open again. She laughed at herself and sniffled. "Silly woman."

Nigel stood there and watched until the SUV was out of sight. He could feel his own eyes get misty and there was no way he was going to let the young airman see him that way, so he took a little time to gather his composure.

When he turned around, Airman Williams had Nigel's bike out of the guard shack. "Here you go, Chief."

"Thank you, Williams."

"You're welcome. You know what, Chief?" The airman nodded his head toward where the SUV had parked. "When I grow up, I want to be just like you."

"Be careful what you ask for, kid. By the way, I'm pulling out of the marina today, so you guys and gals won't have to babysit my bike anymore."

"Where are you going?"

"Home, shipmate. I'm going home."

"Fair winds, Chief."

"And following seas to you, shippie. And hey, when I get back down here, I expect you to be at least a petty officer second class."

"Roger that."

As the diesel engine warmed up, Nigel went around *MisChief* one last time to make sure she was ready and secured for sea. He was inspecting the turnbuckles of his starboard standing rigging when a voice startled him.

"I can't believe you are just up and leaving. This is paradise, man. How can you go?"

Nigel turned his head to find Steve Bailes on the dock holding a Diet Coke. He held up the DC. "Thought I'd bring you a farewell cocktail."

Nigel got up and joined him on the dock. "Thanks, buddy." He gave a quick glance back at this boat and said, "It's just time to go, Steve. I have an old, boring, not-so-glamorous life waiting for me, and I can't wait to get back to it."

Steve handed Nigel the can. "When will you be back?"

"Don't know. But keep my slip open for me."

"Screw you, man. First come, first serve."

"You're such a pal. Thanks for everything, though. Really. The past year has been very therapeutic."

"Not a problem. You leaving now?"

Nigel looked up at the flags. Winds were as forecasted, out of the east northeast. "Now is as good a time as any. Give me a hug."

They did and patted each other on the back.

"Take care buddy," said Nigel. "Will you help cast me off?"

"Sure."

Once the boat was free from the dock, Steve said, "Hey! Does this mean Sylvia Mason is an eligible female again?"

"Shut your hole, Bailes. And don't give it another thought!"

"You're a selfish bastard."

"She's off limits, dammit!" Nigel smiled and waved as he and *MisChief* eased out into the Boca Chica Channel.

Chapter Nineteen

Since Nigel did all the prep work the day before, getting underway was quick and easy. Before Nigel left to meet Sylvia at Blue Heaven, he had already taken care of everything, even diving on the bottom to scrub it clean. He was glad he did, too. While *MisChief's* bottom wasn't badly fouled, it certainly had growth that would have hindered speed and performance. Not anymore.

The channel leading in and out of Boca Chica is relatively straight, but you dare not to stray. There are places where birds can stand, walk, and watch you sail by.

With the autopilot on, Nigel went below, grabbed his phone, connected his Bluetooth to the stereo, and turned on his TuneIn radio app to stream Oyster Radio, WOYS FM 106.5 out of Apalachicola. Soon, Michael Allen's voice came on, finishing up a public service announcement regarding upcoming GED classes to further local adult education in Franklin County. He added a reminder for those in Eastpoint to lock those garbage cans because of an increased presence of bears. Then he reported the local news, weather, and a beach report warning. "Hey, folks, it's a double red flag day on the beaches of St. George Island. That means it is illegal to get into the water. So, unless you want to ruin your vacation by having Sheriff Martin throw you in jail, I'd stay on the sand."

It all placed a smile on Nigel's face. *Familiarity*, he thought. *Now that's what I'm talking about*. Then, once the music started back up, Nigel was sure and solid in his convictions. *Salt in the Blood*, by his buddy Brian

Bowen, came out of the speakers. If that alone wasn't proof positive, nothing could be. When he left St. Joe, Brian had started to date Candice. Nigel wondered if she had kicked him to the curb, too. *Probably*. The thought made him laugh, so he turned up the music.

With the mainsail up, they were motor sailing down the channel. Nigel was in a good place. Once they cleared the channel, Nigel gave himself and *MisChief* plenty of space away from the shoals before heading west toward the main Key West channel. The plan was to give Key West a final flyby, then pick up the northwest channel, leaving Big Mullet Key to port and head out toward the open Gulf of Mexico. It was a good plan until a damn cruise ship began its passage in the channel behind him. Though the ship was still some distance away, Nigel wasted no time getting out of the behemoth's way. *I guess it's a good day to leave after all*; he thought. Overachieving tourons were about to invade the streets and town. If there was one thing his time in Key West taught him, it was to stay clear of Duval Street when the cruise ships disembark their humans on shore.

Out of danger, Nigel made a beeline across the open water to pick up the channel. He was sailing now, though he left the engine running, just in case he needed to engage the screw. With the breeze picking up and still out of the northeast, *MisChief* surged along on close reach toward the channel marker. Once inside, the wind would be on the starboard beam and *MisChief* would really light up the clear, beautiful blue water. Nigel grabbed his Spot X satellite communicator and fired it. When it had connected, he sent a quick text to Red with his position. *On my way!* A couple minutes later, Red replied. *Safe travels buddy. See ya soon!*

Nigel replied, *Going as fast as the old girl will deliver! Ha!*

Nigel put the Spot X away and settled down in the cockpit. Then his phone rang. He looked down at the number. It had a 202 area code. He thought about it. *Two oh two. Isn't that a D.C. area code?* He let it go to voicemail. Moments later, the notification light flashed to show a message. *Knock yourself out, fella. This fish ain't biting.*

After several minutes, his phone bonged with a text message. He opened the text and looked at the screen. It was the same 202 area code again. The message read: *Call me.*

Bong!

Please.

Bong!

It's Desi.

It took all of two seconds for the name to register in his brain. Desi is short for Desiderio. Last name Machado. It was a name he wasn't expecting to think about, but given recent developments, it made sense. Desi is an operative within the Cuban Embassy in Washington, D.C. Truth be told, Desi's loyalties are not to his homeland, at least the one that exists today. More importantly, he works closely with Basilio and his work against the regime.

Nigel felt his heart sink. *I know I'm going to resent this.* He was about to press the dial button, but stopped. "No, dammit. I'm done."

A little while longer. *Bong*!

Please.

Nigel closed his eyes and squinted hard. One of Nigel's greatest traits, and perhaps weakness, is his loyalty to his friends. So much so that he is often... *loyal to a fault*. He opened his eyes, pressed dial, and put the phone to his ear.

"Chief. Thank you for calling me back. It has been a long time."

"Yes, it has. And to be honest, I can't say I'm thrilled you're calling. I'm underway at the moment. I'm headed home. You remember. Port St. Joe."

"Yes, I do, but please, Basilio needs your help."

"I'm sure Basilio Valdez has enough resources that he can pull off whatever he has planned without me. You could say that I've started my second retirement. Please send him my best wishes."

Nigel saw the red channel marker in the distance and adjusted his steering, the sails, and the autopilot.

"Please, Chief. Hear me out."

"I'll listen, but I can't guarantee how long I remain in cell phone coverage."

"I'll be brief then. They didn't just kill Dr. Cabrera. It was an execution in a graveyard. A bullet to the back of his head. They did the same to the other guy. The other guy's name was Carlos Torres. He's... was a taxi driver and a good friend of the resistance. Carlos had taken Dr. Cabrera to his father-in-law's house. They were to collect his two lovely children, Lucia and Antonio, and escape."

"So, what happened?" asked Nigel with a slight cringe.

For the same reason Nigel cringed, Desi grinned. Nigel's question meant he was taking interest.

"Basilio is still learning more, but he is sure that MININT is involved. That's the Ministry of..."

"I know what MININT is. Basilio explained it to me. But why would they kill him, anyway?"

"Because they are brutal sons of bitches. And that is being polite. God reserves a special place in hell for each of them."

As he listened, *MisChief* entered the northwest channel, and he adjusted for course and sail trim.

"Yes. Once MININT learned that Dr. Cabrera escaped his post in Venezuela, we believe they paid her father a visit."

"Desi... why are you and not Basilio telling me all this?"

Desi said nothing.

"Desssiiiiii? Where is Basilio?"

"He's planning his return to Cuba."

"Where is he?"

"I'd rather not say."

"Going back to Cuba. Isn't that a bit dangerous?"

"Yes, when you are on the regime's most wanted list, it isn't wise to return. But he feels it is necessary."

"What's he planning to do?"

"To learn more and visit Dr. Benita's father if necessary."

Nigel said nothing. *Oh shit.*

"He needs your help, Nigel."

"No, he doesn't. Y'all have plenty in your camp to do whatever needs to be done."

"Yes, and they are all Cuban. Basilio needs you, a gringo. A gringo with your special talents."

"Dammit, Desi."

"Like he's already told you. He needs you in Belize."

Nigel said nothing.

"Basilio would be forever grateful. Not to mention, once everything is done, and the word gets out, you will be a hero to those within the dissident movement."

"I'm tired of being a hero, Desi."

Desi said nothing as Nigel thought about Basilio. His old friend that he hadn't seen or heard from for years and years, and now, suddenly, he was back in Nigel's life. And while many years had passed since he and Basilio shared dangerous endeavors, it felt like only yesterday. He thought of Dr. Benita and the kindness she showed him despite the pain she endured. He thought of her husband. Another doctor. A man he would never know, and how monsters pressed a muzzle to the back of his head and pulled the trigger. All because his love for his children was greater than his devotion and dedication to his corrupt country. Then there were the children. He couldn't remember their names, but it didn't matter. In a sense, they were being held hostage. Trapped, just like their loving mother and their father who *they* took from this world. Now Basilio is heading into the storm.

"Shit, Desi. He can't go back to Cuba. I'll go." The words just came right out of his mouth. He wasn't expecting to hear them, but they did. "I'll go. I don't even know what he has planned, but I'll do it."

"No, Chief. He must go. The betrayal and execution of Dr. Cabrera are now very personal, and he must handle things in the homeland. He will be fine, but does this mean you will now go to Belize?"

Nigel looked ahead. The end of the channel was near. He was about to enter the vast navigable waters of the Gulf of Mexico. There he would bring *MisChief* hard on the wind and point her more north than northwest. *Dammit!* Nigel threw the helm over and tacked the boat to head back toward Key West and Boca Chica. "What does he need for me to do?"

Chapter Twenty

"What do you mean you're not leaving?" asked Dan. The harbormaster took off the cap he was wearing and pulled at his hair. "I've already left a message for the next guy on the waiting list that the slip was available. That's messed up."

"Damn, Dan, you didn't waste any time, did you? Who is it?"

"Some Lieutenant JG, named Swanson."

"Ah, he's just a JO. A junior officer that doesn't know shit. Tell him, 'Chief Logan changed his mind, and he's keeping the slip.'"

"He's going to be pissed. He's been waiting for months now."

"He'll get over it, and it won't be the last time he feels the sting of disappointment."

"Why the change of heart? You seemed mighty determined to get back home."

"I still am. I forgot that I have a follow-up doctor's appointment."

"Well, crap!"

"What is it?" asked Nigel.

"A certain Lieutenant Swanson just walked into the office building."

"Ha! Sorry about that. Good luck."

"You owe me."

Nigel grinned and scattered his words. "Wha... sa... Dan. Did... cat... tha... Com... gain?"

"You heard me, dammit!"

Nigel ended the call.

"Logan! I'm talking to you!"

"Harbormaster, Dan?"

He looked up to find the young man standing at his desk. The JG stood in his pressed khakis. A uniform that adds the look of maturity to anyone who wears it. With Swanson, the look of maturity was undermined by his fresh pimples, rosy cheeks, and red hair. Dan acted like he couldn't remember him. "Can I help you with something?"

"I'm Lieutenant Mark Swanson. You called about my slip."

"Oh... yeah... well, have a seat."

Steve Bailes had his back to the bar as he loaded beers into one of the chest refrigerators as Nigel entered Navigator's. "Hey there, pal. I'll take a Diet Coke when you get a free minute."

Steve stood with a dropped jaw as he recognized the voice and saw Nigel's reflection in the mirror. He turned around. "What in the world are you doing back here?"

"I came back. It was a quick visit home."

Steve stretched his neck and looked over Nigel's shoulder to see *Mis-Chief* back in her slip. "Well, you have a problem, pal. Dan has already reassigned your slip to some JG. He was in here earlier, checking it out before going to see Dan."

"I know. That's all been taken care of. He's been told he'll need to wait a little longer."

"That won't make him happy. He was pretty excited when he left."

"What kind of boat does he have?"

"A Bayliner. Some old cabin cruiser."

"Yuck."

"Yeah. Really, though, why are you back?"

"Long story. Hopefully, it's just temporary, and I can be on my way. Then the JO can move in and dress the place up with his piece of shit cruiser. Change of subject. Have you gotten around to listing my bike on the book of faces marketplace?"

Steve slid Nigel a DC. "Noooo. For crying out loud, you just left a few hours ago. I have more things to worry about around here than to waste time selling your goofy bike."

"Good. I need the goofy thing to ride into town."

Nigel leaned the bike up against the fence and took the key. As he had peddled through town, he wondered how stupid it looked for one person to be on a bike built for two. The thought came and went just as quick, because deep down... he didn't care. However, the bike made him think of Sylvia since the empty seat was hers. Though she bitched about it, he knew she enjoyed riding. Note: riding, not pedaling.

It was already dark when he arrived, and as usual, the old metal gate squealed to announce somebody on the marina dock. Two familiar beauties came out on the forward deck of their houseboat. One called out, "Well hello, Mr. Logan."

"Evening, Stacy." He nodded to the other. "Same to you, Ms. Barbie. And how many times do I have to tell y'all to call me Chief?"

As the ladies giggled, Nigel looked down the dock, saw what he was looking for, and said, "Well, I see the boat bum is in. Ladies, if you will excuse me."

Cam saw Nigel talking with Stacy and Barbie and threw up a wave when their eyes met. As Nigel came down the dock, Cam's dog Walter jumped from the boat and hurried to greet him: tail wagging, mouth open, tongue and ears flopping from side to side.

Nigel bent over to receive his welcoming committee and Walter hit him hard enough to sock Nigel back on his ass. "Damn, boy. Are you happy to see me or what?" He grabbed and rubbed the dog's ears. "Is the old man home?" Nigel got to his feet. "Come on, let's go find out."

Walter ran ahead, and Nigel followed.

"Sorry about that," Cam said as Nigel got close enough to hear.

"Not a problem. A friend back home has an old goat named Maxine. When she playfully lays into you, it isn't pretty."

"Speaking of home. I thought you were gone."

"Change of plans. Hopefully not for long. May I come aboard?"

"Sure. Can I get you a diet?"

"Well, actually..." Nigel pointed with his nose toward Cam's glass he was holding. "I gather that's a Wild Turkey?"

Cam raised his glass up and looked at what remained in his ice cubes. "You know it."

"I think I'll have one of those."

"Oh, shit. Really?"

"Yeah."

"Have a seat."

As Cam walked away, Nigel watched him leave. "Where's Diane?"

"She's working late, so I have to make my own drinks."

Moments later, Cam handed Nigel his bourbon.

"She spoils the hell out of you, Mr. Derringer!"

"I know. It's easy to get used to, but don't go hating. For some reason..." Cam scratched at his chin. "I can't recall the last time a rich and beautiful woman flew me to Belize for an intimate getaway on a private island."

"Funny you bring that up?"

"What?"

"Belize."

"What about it?"

Nigel took a long sip from his drink. The burn of the booze was tasty and warmed his throat as he swallowed, but it took his breath away as he said, "How much gas does it take to get there?"

Chapter Twenty-One

"You need me to take you to Belize? Again?"

"Yes."

"It was so good the first time that you and Sylvia just can't stay away?"

"It was great the first time, but Sylvia isn't going?"

"Oh!"

Nigel told Cam everything. He left nothing off the table. That wouldn't have been fair. Cam is a private eye. He runs into a little trouble from time to time, so he's used to it. However, Nigel wanted Cam to know everything so he could make up his own mind.

"So you just need me to take you?"

"And pick me up when the time is right."

"And when I pick you up, you will have this doctor woman with you? A Cuban national with no passport."

"Yes. That is correct, or at least that's the plan."

"And we are going to reunite this woman with her two children. And these kids are currently in Cuba?"

"Yes, and again... that's the plan."

"So, just to be clear. We're smuggling Cubans into the U.S."

"Smuggling is such an ugly word. I've learned to think of it as *exporting and importing*. It's a much more pleasant way of expressing it."

"What if this woman doesn't cooperate?"

"She will."

"How do you know?"

"I don't."

"Humph! That's what I thought."

"And how do we get her out without a passport?"

Behind a coy smile, Nigel said, "We bypass immigration." Nigel saw the look of uncertainty grow on Cam's face. "Listen, buddy. You do not have to do this. No problem, really."

Cam got up, walked back inside his boat, and returned with the bottle. He recharged his and Nigel's glasses and sat back down. He took a good long sip and said, "And your Cuban buddy, this Basilio guy, you say he's picking up the tab?"

"All of it."

Cam took another pull from his drink and said, "Dammit, Nigel. What's the plan again?"

Two days later, Nigel leaned his bike against a wall at the Geiger Key Marina and Smokehouse. He went inside and grabbed a picnic table by the water and sat so he could see who came and went. After a few minutes, he looked at his watch. It read 1307. A couple of minutes later, the bartender brought him another Diet Coke, and as he stepped away, Nigel saw a familiar face and an unknown associate enter the bar. Nigel stood and waited for them to join him. "You're late," he said aloud. Nigel reached out his hand, and the men shook. "Desi. Good to see you again. I think. Who is your friend?"

"We'll call him Marco, if that's okay with you."

Nigel turned loose of Desi's hand and extended it to Marco. He took it and Nigel said, "Nice to meet you, Marco. I'm Mary Poppins. Please... both of you, take a seat."

"This place is like you mentioned," said Desi. "Off the beaten path."

"It's quiet and very local, and the mentality is simple: Stay out of my business and I'll stay out of yours. Once we finish here and part ways, it will be like we were never here."

"Excellent."

"So, where are we at? And how is Basilio coming along?"

"Basilio is just fine. He is now in the country. Staying at a safe house outside of Cienfuegos City. He'll stay there until he hears from you in Placencia."

"How am I supposed to do that?"

Desi looked at Marco and nodded.

Marco produced a bag and slid it across the table.

Nigel slowly took possession of it, put it under the table on his lap, and gave Desi an inquiring stare.

"It's money. Cash for you and your pilot friend. A combination of American and Belize dollars. There should be more than enough to hold you over. There is also an Iridium satellite phone. It's activated, so it is ready to go. Basilio has one just like it. His number is in there, along with some notes that may help along the way. He wishes to hear from you once you've observed the doctor for a couple of days."

Nigel watched as Marco got up and left.

"That's it?"

"Pretty much," said Desi. "There isn't much more we can discuss. It will be up to you and Basilio to work out the rest."

And with that, Desi and Nigel stood and shook hands. Nigel remained standing. Once Desi was gone, he opened the bag for a quick look. "Damn," he said to himself. *That should cover it.*

Chapter Twenty-Two

Approximately three hundred-sixty-five miles away, and at the precise moment Nigel mounted his bike, the door of the City Bar opened. Luke McKenzie and his goat, Maxine, walked in. Maxine took off in search of her buddy, Daisy, the bar dog. As usual, Maxine found her sleeping under stool seventeen. Luke made a beeline for the bar. When he saddled a stool, Candice, the manager-bartender, placed a draft in front of him. "Howdy, Luke."

He took a sip. "Hmmm. Good." He looked at Candice. "Have you heard anything further?"

"About?" she lied.

"You know damn well what I'm talking about. Nigel. Any word on when he'll be getting back?"

She rolled her eyes. "It's a sailboat, Luke. Not exactly a cigarette boat and it's only been a few days since he left the Keys."

Luke said nothing.

"And if there is one thing I've learned about that boat, it rarely goes straight to where you are going. Depending on the wind, if there is any, there's a lot of zigging and zagging going on. He calls it tacking."

"Well, it's been what? Three days now? It shouldn't be too much longer. He needs to hurry. I want to see the young punk, and I won't live forever."

"Hush your mouth, old man. Stop talking like that. You may be ninety-five, but you're doing better than most that were born the same year."

"HEY! Don't put years on me. I'm only..."

Another voice behind the bar piped up. "Well, I can't wait to see him, either. That's for sure."

Candice cut her bar-help with a look. "Oh, yeah. And why might that be, Tara?"

Tara Appleton and Nigel were once good for each other when they both needed it the most. Tara had found herself in a terrible relationship, over in Eastpoint. It was with a drug dealer and she had zero opportunity to run. At the same time, Nigel struggled to get his act together. Too much booze and self-pity. The breakup with Candice sent him in a spiral. It was unintentional and unexpected, but Nigel, under false pretenses, ended up saving Tara. And Tara, in many ways, helped return the favor.

The intimacies he and Tara shared were brief, but they were sweet and innocent and welcomed by both parties. And while Tara knows the history between Nigel and her boss, Candice knows nothing of the brief relationship enjoyed by Tara and her ex. However, she has always had her suspicions. Especially when Nigel so willingly let Tara stay at his cottage while he was away. And then... there was that kiss.

The look Candice gave Tara wasn't much different from the look she gave her just over a year ago. It was the last time Nigel was in the bar. Nigel knew it was time to leave. Time to get away and continue his efforts to screw his head on straight.

They held a big gathering at the bar to send him off. When it was time to go, he went around the room gathering goodbye sugars from all the gals. All except one. Candice refused and kept her back turned most of the time, but... in the mirror behind the bar, she caught Tara more than making up for it. While it wasn't overly passionate, it was intimate enough to lift more than a few eyebrows in the room, including Candice's. Especially since, to her knowledge, Tara and Nigel had just met minutes earlier. She thought, *What the hell?*

"Excuse me?" asked Tara.

"Why would you be so excited to see him? You don't even know him. Right?"

"Ah, well... I don't know. He is my landlord. And he seems so nice when we communicate."

"You two communicate?"

"Well, sure. When I have questions about the cottage and stuff."

"Uh, huh?"

"I'm sorry Candice. Is there something wrong? Did I do something?"

"I don't know Tara. Did you?"

"I can't imagine what. I'm not even sure what we are talking about."

The entire time the exchange between Candice and Tara volleyed back and forth, Luke's eyes bounced back and forth as he sipped his beer. A shit-eating grin grew on his face when he interrupted the banter. "Are we about to have a little catfight? I love a good catfight."

Candice turned her attention toward him. "Oh, shut up, Luke. No, there won't be a fight."

"Well, damn then," he said.

Ready to change the focus, Tara asked, "Are you ready for another round?"

Luke said nothing. He emptied his pint glass, brought it down on the bar, and gave it a little slide toward her.

"Coming right up," she said, and all the tension in the room disappeared.

Later, after a few more beers, Luke wagged a finger for Candice to come over.

She did. "What is it, Luke?"

"You still love him, don't you?"

"What are you talking about?"

Luke shook his head. "Remind me to never ask you to lie for me. You suck at it."

Candice said nothing.

"Sugar. Look who you are talking to."

She cast a glance at him and saw those old, comforting eyes she had confided in so many times over the years.

"He's been gone for over a year now," he said. "You were in love with him when he left, though you wouldn't admit it, and you're still in love with him today. Own up to it."

"Even if I do, it changes nothing. He's still Nigel Logan, and it sickens me to worry about him and his endeavors all the time. It's best I just pretend he never existed. But so much for that idea. Just when I was getting close to convincing myself that he was just a dream, Trixie and Red came barging in to announce his return. My stomach has been upside down ever since."

"Have you given any thought to the idea that he isn't the same? He may have settled down like he promised. That he would stay away from trouble and live a normal life. That's all he ever wanted, you know, a normal life with you."

"Well, Luke... it's like you said, 'He's been gone over a year now.' Even if I were interested, and I'm not, I'm sure he's moved on by now."

"Do you really believe that girl? Come on!"

Candice stood up straight in an act of defiance and slapped the bar. "Tara! Luke is cut off. He's had enough to drink. He's talking out of his head." Then she stormed off to the back storeroom.

Tara looked at Luke and watched him wink and mouth the words. *It's okay. I'll have one more.*

Tara returned a grin and pulled a fresh beer from the draft station.

Meanwhile, Candice sat on a case of Jim Beam and privately broke down into tears. Tears of excitement. Excitement she had been trying to ignore. But the urge was too strong. She couldn't stand it any longer and she smiled. Nigel was coming home. Time would tell if it were a good thing.

Chapter Twenty-Three

The next afternoon Nigel and Cam sat on the deck of Cam's boat.

"Why can't I just fly you into Belize City?"

"Desi said it would be best to stay off the radar of Belize immigration if possible. If things went sideways with Basilio, it would only be a matter of time before the Cuban Embassy would check with immigration and know I was in the country. And vice versa, if I am caught helping Dr. Cabrera, they would immediately suspect Basilio was involved in some way."

"Why would the Cubans give a rat's ass about Nigel Logan?"

"Well, let's just say that several years back, when I first met Basilio, I sort of made a name for myself with the Cuban Embassy in D.C. and the regime in Havana. I got caught up in Basilio's dissident resistance. They led me to believe they had assassinated Basilio, and I didn't take it too well. I called, harassed, and threatened the hell out of them. Almost every day. So much so that… Let's just say I'm pretty sure I'm part of Basilio's permanent record."

"This is great. Not only are you asking me to smuggle a Cuban out of Belize, but now I'm going to smuggle you in and out of Belize."

"Cam, please… import and export. Don't make matters worse than they really are."

"Diane will not like this at all."

"So, you haven't said anything yet?"

"No. I wanted to know more first."

"We'll only be gone for a few days. It might be best to not say anything."

Cam became visibly irritated. "That's enough, Logan! Diane and I hide nothing from each other. Do you understand me?"

Nigel bowed and ducked his head and held up his palms in surrender. "Sorry, Cam." He lifted his head slightly to make eye contact. "Really. I mean it."

"Sorry I yelled," said Cam. "It's just Diane and I are a team, solid as a rock. And we might need her. Let's say something does go sideways. She is smart. It's a good idea that she knows everything so she can act."

"You're right."

"So, tell me about this old airfield."

Nigel pulled out a chart. And found the spot. "Here it is. Desi said it was an old, abandoned airport. It just sits there. Runway is still in pretty good shape. He said the embassy in Belize City uses it from time to time when they are not looking to draw attention."

"And after I drop you off, I fly on into Belize City?"

"Yes. And wait. Grab a nice room, hang out, see the sights, be a tourist. If you don't hear from me within five days, get on your plane, fly home to Key West, give Diane a kiss for me, and forget you ever knew me."

Cam scrunched his eyebrows. "I don't like the sound of that."

"I'm serious, but don't worry. You'll hear from me."

"How can I be so sure?" asked Cam, as his face tightened with confusion.

"Because I'm Nigel Logan. Isn't that enough?"

Cam rolled his eyes. "And we leave in the morning?"

"Yup. You just fly the plane and leave the nasty crap to me. I'll meet you at the plane at seven. Right now, I need to get some rest."

As Nigel stood and turned to leave, Cam asked, "Why are you doing this?"

Nigel stopped and turned around. "Why are you?"

"I guess because I have a few screws loose."

"Well, that's reason enough for me, too. Thanks, Cam."

As Nigel walked up the dock, Diane came through the gate and they both stopped.

"Afternoon, Nigel."

Nigel nodded his head, then leaned in for a kiss on the cheek. "Diane. Good to see you."

She looked past him to Cam, who was waving from the deck. "Have you and Dad been plotting to save the world?"

"No, not the entire world. Just one family at a time."

Diane lifted her forehead and gave a little shake. "What is that supposed to mean?"

Nigel turned to look at Cam, then back to her. "You'll find out soon enough." He pretended to tip a hat, and before walking away said, "Have a pleasant evening, Diane."

She watched Nigel go out the gate. Then she turned and found Cam standing with his hands on his hips.

Chapter Twenty-Four

It was late. After midnight. Basilio and two other men watched as another stood, peeking out the blinds of a window.

"Carlito. Do you see him?" asked Basilio.

"Not yet."

"Do you see anything else?" asked another man named Emilio.

Carlito turned to the group. "Luckily, no." He returned his attention to the street. "Wait! Yes. Here he comes. Emilio. Get the door."

He did, and another man quickly ducked inside. Emilio closed and locked the door. Then he and the man embraced. "Good to see you, Javiero."

"Same here, my friend."

"And you were not followed?"

"I wouldn't have come to the house if I thought so."

Miguel, the other man with Basilio, said, "See anything, Carlito?"

Carlito kept his focus on the street. Nothing moved. "I think we are good." He turned to face the group. "We're okay."

"Then let's get started," said Miguel.

All those in opposition to the Cuban regime are considered enemies of the state. There is no freedom of speech or expression, so whenever active members of the resistance want to meet to discuss the dissident movement, they must do so in secret. They keep their activities underground to avoid long prison sentences.

Not all who are against the oppressive government are active in the movement. They live as their government demands, by intimidation and fear. They dare not speak out, attend secretive meetings, or attend public protests. Who could blame them? They are the silent majority, but they revere those willing to be brave and further the cause of freedom. These brave souls are heroes, such as the Cienfuegos Fire of Freedom, the men meeting in the home of Carlito Sanchez. Together, they risk everything to discuss, plan, and execute small initiatives to undermine the state leadership. They understand power is found in numbers, and carefully identifying and collecting other brave, like-minded countrymen is a priority.

Then there are the foolish dissidents who plot and openly protest against the government in the streets. While they openly display their displeasure and garner plenty of attention, they cannot recognize their actions change nothing, except to identify themselves as traitors worthy of being caged behind bars. One can oppose violations of human rights, but little can be done if you are sitting in prison.

In the home of Carlito, there would be no discussions on recruitment. They focused on Basilio and his concerns.

Miguel and Basilio stood around a table as the others joined them.

"Please, Javiero, come. We have someone we want you to meet."

Basilio extended his hand as Javiero closed in.

"This is Basilio Valdez of Miami, formerly from Batabano."

"Miami?" said Javiero as he took Basilio's hand.

"He is staying with me for a few days," said Carlito, "until..."

Javiero's brow lifted.

"Until I'm ready to make a move," said Basilio.

"Please, everyone," said Carlito, "take a seat."

They did.

"So, Carlito," said Javiero, "since he is staying with you. I'm guessing the authorities are unaware of his homecoming."

"That would be correct," said Basilio.

"Interesting. What is all this about?"

"Basilio," said Carlito, "please tell Javiero why you are here."

"I am here on behalf of Alejandro and Benita Cabrera."

Javiero's eyes opened wide and darted around the room at all the other men. "Alejandro is dead."

Basilio nodded. "I am aware of that. It was more of an execution. Miguel tells me you may have some information about what happened."

Javiero looked at Miguel.

"He is okay, Javiero. I've told him a little, but thought it best if he heard it from you."

Javiero nodded his head in agreement.

"Gracias, Javiero," said Basilio. "I'm interested to hear what you have to say."

Javiero started, "I am a barber here in Palmira. In the eyes of many, I am hated, since I am known as being loyal to our most corrupt and disgusting government. And while I have customers who support the resistance, many of the heads I cut are deeply devoted to the government. I have earned their trust, so when they talk… I listen."

"What have you heard?"

Javiero lowered his head and spoke to the table. "Alejandro and Benita are so beloved in these parts. They are skilled doctors and surely missed." He got quiet for a spell, then said, "I wasn't expecting to hear what I heard, and I almost lost control of my cover. I wanted to slice that old man's throat. It would have only taken a second. Sparing him took all the strength I could muster."

"What?" said Basilio. "Please tell me."

Javiero raised his head and looked Basilio in the eye. "It was Benita's father, Fredrico. He was the one to call MININT and turn Alejandro in."

"His own father-in-law?"

"Si."

"How do you know this?"

"He told me, himself. He was in my chair, getting a shave. It was a couple of days after they found Alejandro. I asked him about it. He told me how Alejandro came to the house and how he called Garcia. They arrived moments later and apprehended Alejandro. I shook in anger. He had his head back and eyes closed as he spoke. I had the straight razor placed under his chin and tilted enough to make a clean cut back behind his ear. Oh… how I wanted to do it, but I had a shop full of customers."

"Garcia?"

"Si. Colonel Garcia. He is the regional head of the local MININT division. A bad actor. Often takes matters into his own hands. The regime loves him because he is successful in maintaining…" He used fingers to make air quotes, '*proper social order*.' "If the citizens are quietly scared, behaved, and unwilling to promote havoc, he has done his job."

"I understand he, Alejandro, had planned to collect his children and run."

"Si. They were going to pick up a boat and sneak out of the country."

"There was another man killed with Alejandro."

All the other men around the table lowered their heads in a subtle tribute to their old friend.

"His name was Carlos," said Carlito. "He was one of us and a taxi driver. He was helping Alejandro with transportation."

"Did Fredrico sound happy that his son-in-law was dead?"

"No, not exactly. Even he said that he didn't expect that to happen. A long prison sentence maybe, but not that."

"What else did he say?"

Javiero shrugged. "That it was Alejandro's fault. He said that Alejandro should have been more loyal."

"And the children?"

"They are still with Fredrico."

"I think I need to meet this family traitor. Where can I find him?"

"At Parque de Palmira. He is there almost every day, playing dominoes and drinking rum with his comrades."

"And I gather we know where he lives?"

All the other men nodded.

"Javiero, will you have time tomorrow to partner with this steadfast loyalist in a few games of dominoes?"

The men around the table smiled.

"Basilio, my new friend, it would be an honor."

Chapter Twenty-Five

The next morning, Cam walked around his plane doing his pre-flight check as Diane held firm to her opinions. "I don't like this, Mr. Logan. Not one bit."

"Please, don't call me that, and I know. He said you wouldn't be crazy about it all."

"He's not crazy about the whole thing, either. You know that, right? I asked him why he was doing it then, and he couldn't come up with a suitable answer. He said, 'I'm not really sure, but I feel like I need to.' I've never known him to do anything he wasn't sure about. It scares me."

Nigel looked over at Cam as he checked the tires and landing gear. "I understand, and I don't want to cause a rift between you two."

Diane said nothing.

Nigel turned toward her. "I mean it. I'll tell him to forget it. He doesn't have to do it. I'll make other plans."

"You would do that?"

"Absolutely. I'm not looking for him to do something he's not sure of. Trust me, I need him to be sure. In my line of business, confidence is paramount."

"Your line of business?"

Even Nigel couldn't believe he used those words. However, in the back of his mind, he understood why. Then he lied, "It is just an expression. That's all."

"Hey! Nigel," yelled Cam. "It's time to go. Come on."

Nigel looked at Diane. “I promise. I’ll tell him.”

She nodded her head.

Nigel started toward the plane. He saw Cam climbing aboard, so he threw up his hand. “Cam! Hold up.”

Diane watched as Nigel spoke with him. Cam stood with his arms crossed and Nigel became animated, using his hands in expression and once turning to point at Diane. After the exchange of words, Nigel turned to look at Diane. Then he slowly went aboard as Cam slowly walked over to Diane. Once there, he kissed her on the cheek.

“I’ll be fine, dear. Don’t worry.”

“That’s fine, dandy, and easy for you to say.”

He took her in his arms. “Listen. I’m sure I want to do this. Really.”

“Why?”

He gave a little laugh and said, “This is going to sound stupid.”

“Try me.”

“Because he’s Nigel Logan.”

“What the hell is that supposed to mean?”

“I wish I knew.”

She said nothing.

“Hold the fort down for the next few days. I’ll let you know when I’m coming home, and I’ll expect an ample supply of honey buns and Wild Turkey to celebrate our return. Got it?”

She returned a not-so-confident smile and nodded.

Moments later, Cam climbed aboard, started forward to the cockpit, and stopped. “You’re in my seat. Scoot over.”

Nigel turned back to look. “I was thinking I would fly. I’m a quick learner.”

“Right now... move your ass.”

He did, and Cam climbed into the left seat.

“One more time, Cam. You don’t have to do this?”

“One more time. Yes, I do. Now buckle up.”

“Buckle up in a plane. I’ve never quite understood the reason.”

“It’s so they can find the bodies.”

“Nice. Very reassuring.”

“Just buckle up.”

The park was stirring with activity as the noontime light warmed the air. Javiero and Basilio slowly approached from a distance.

"There they are, Basilio. The one facing you from the other side of the table is Fredrico."

As they neared, a cacophony of excitement came from the table.

Cuban dominoes is not a passive game of relaxation. It is a spirited team competition, falling just short of being considered a contact sport. Two on two, and highly animated, full of smack talk and table slapping as the tiles meet the tabletop and the bottle of rum is passed around. Basilio studied the old man as they approached. For his age, he was quick, agile, and smart with the tongue. He was impressed, but that was as far as his admiration would extend. The old man was still an enemy of his country's people. That was something Basilio would not forget.

Once close enough, Javiero stopped and grabbed Basilio's arm. "Hold on."

"What?"

Javiero turned away so as not to be heard. Basilio followed. "This could be good. The man playing with Fredrico. He is like me, a counterfeit loyalist. His name is Riel Serrano. He is a local automotive mechanic. He has a shop across town where he serves the community and some vehicles of MININT."

"MININT?"

"Si. He has earned their trust."

"And I gather you both are familiar with one another."

Javiero nodded and turned back toward the game.

"And what about the other two?" asked Basilio.

"They are the real thing. Both worked for the regime but are now retired."

"So, we are pulling for the bastards to lose."

"Si. Then it will be three against one. But..."

"What?"

"Over there. On the bench. There is another team looking to join the table."

Basilio kept an eye on the rum bottle. It was getting low. He looked around and nudged Javiero on the arm. "I'll be right back."

A few minutes later, he returned. "How is it looking?"

"It is close. Riel has one tile left. Fredrico, two. The bastards have five collectively." As the ruckus continued around the table, Riel made a fist with his right, which contained his last tile and knocked rapidly on the table with great excitement as he maintained eye contact with Fredrico.

Fredrico looked away from Riel's eyes and looked at the table and his remaining tiles. He only had one play on the table. A three. When he picked up his three-two tile, he saw Riel stand, shaking his fist in the air. Fredrico slammed the tile down and grabbed the rum. Riel's attention turned to his opponent on the left. He could tell in an instant he didn't have a tile to play and didn't wait for him to pass. Riel opened his fist and slammed his double two tile down on Fredrico's play, and exclaimed, "Finito!"

Fredrico reached across the table and offered the bottle. Riel took it and downed what remained. There was no need to count the pips on their opponent's tiles. Victory. The two bastards slammed the table. Domino tiles jumped and scattered about, then they pushed away from the table.

Jeering and laughter continued as Riel collected the tiles and turned them face down for a fresh mixing. As he shuffled the tiles around, he looked up to see who was next and smiled when he saw the next team approach from the bench. Then he saw Javiero with a stranger approaching.

One of the other two called out. "Javiero. Not this game. We are next."

Basilio spoke up. "I'm not so sure about that, as you come empty-handed."

"And who do you think you are?"

Basilio raised his left hand, holding a fresh bottle of rum. "Call me... Havana Club. Perhaps you have heard of me."

"OH!" said Riel. "That changes everything. Javiero... you and your friend take a seat and prepare to be smacked back to your mommas."

As they sat down, Basilio handed the bottle to Fredrico, as the other two huffed, puffed, and walked away in search of another table.

"Gracias," said Fredrico with a rum-influenced smile. "I am Fredrico and across from me is Riel. What is your name, amigo?"

"Juan," said Basilio. "Juan Valdez from Batabano Bay."

Fredrico gave Basilio a humorous stare, and Riel gave out a boisterous laugh.

"Yes, I know," said Basilio. "It was a cruel joke made by my parents. I've lived with it my entire life."

"Batabano Bay? Sponge harvesters?"

"Yes, my grandfather. But that was in the old days."

As Basilio and Fredrico made small talk, Javiero gave a wink and exchanged confirming glances with Riel.

"Let's go," announced Riel. "Collect your tiles."

"Open that bottle first," Javiero demanded, "and we'll raise a toast to Castro and the ass beating the two of you are about to suffer."

The bottle moved around the table in a counterclockwise manner, just as when playing the game. When the bottle got back to Basilio, he took a small sip, replaced the cork and slammed it down on the table. "Battle."

They each collected their seven tiles, studied them, and arranged them in their preferred order, as Riel gave the instructions. "Playing to two hundred points. Standard play. Scores are rounded up or down accordingly. Who has the spinner?"

Javiero selected the double six tile and slammed it in the middle of the table to start the round. From there, the high jinks commenced.

Riel sat to Javiero's right and was next. He wasted no time getting rid of his six-five tile. Nobody wants to get caught with eleven pips at the end of the round. As the round proceeded, Riel glanced at Javiero, wondering what he had in mind with this stranger who he presumed wasn't named Juan.

Basilio smacked a six-three tile down. "Ha! Do something with that!" He grabbed the bottle and pretended to drink.

"Joder. Tu gilipollas!" yelled Fredrico with a slur. *Fuck. You shithead.* Then tapped the table to pass. He had no play.

Javiero popped a double five on the table and looked up to see Basilio reaching over with the bottle. He took it and drank.

Riel slammed a three-four tile down. "Take that!"

And that is how things progressed for a couple more rounds. Slamming tiles followed by friendly insults, which meant nothing in the actual sense. It was all in competitive fun. The tiles came down fast and furious. The next time Javiero made a play, he said, "Y'all are as good as dead. Like Alejandro!"

Immediately, the game paused.

Catching on to Javiero's intentions, Riel made his play and asked, "Dr. Cabrera?"

Basilio paused and took the game off of its pace. "Who is this Dr. Cabrera?"

Fredrico said nothing, and an eerie quiet took over the table.

"Nobody. Not anymore," said Riel. "A treasonous deserter. Isn't that right, Fredrico?"

Fredrico grabbed the bottle and took a long drink. When he put the rum down, he said, "Callarse la boca!" *Shut your mouth.* "I wish not to discuss it."

Javiero ignored him and explained it to Basilio. "Juan, he was resistant to the ways of our country. A traitor. Fredrico's son-in-law. He is not a problem now. Thanks to Fredrico here."

Fredrico, having already enjoyed too much rum, grabbed the bottle and again yelled, "CALLARSE LA BOCA!" and took another long drink. He slammed the bottle down and lowered his head. "Jugar!" *Play!*

"Fredrico is right," said Basilio and played a four-three tile.

It was now Fredrico's play, and all he did was sway back and forth, gazing through the table, seeing nothing.

"But Fredrico," said Riel in a lower tone, "you did the right thing and honored your homeland. You are a hero."

After hearing that, Fredrico raised his head, took another drink from the bottle, and set it down. It fell over, and he pushed away from the table. "No mas!"

Javiero grabbed the bottle and the three of them watched as Fredrico got up, fell to the ground, and slowly got up and staggered away. Game over.

Chapter Twenty-Six

They again topped off with fuel in Cancun. The registered flight plan had Cam's Cessna heading to Guatemala, so flying over Belize air space would prove nothing out of the ordinary. It was a clear day. The visibility was excellent, maybe too excellent.

"The countryside is beautiful," said Nigel.

Cam opened his eyes, tilted his head, and looked out the window. "Yes, it is. Lush and green."

"Are we over Belize yet?"

"Yes. We'll be over Belize City in about twenty minutes." He pulled out his phone to look at the map and the airstrip's location again. He zoomed in to study the satellite imagery. "And you said this Desi guy says this is a good runway?"

"That's what he said."

Cam squinted at the screen in hopes it would help his focus. It never works. He put the phone away. "Well... I guess we'll find out in about forty-five minutes."

They flew in silence. Nigel rested, hoping to get ahead of some sleep. He did that for most of the trip. Rest when you can. There's no guarantee there will be time in the future. He never felt the plane as it started its descent, but when it made a hard left bank, his eyes popped open. "Where are we?"

"Over the field. I want a good look at it."

Nigel looked over Cam's shoulder as the plane circled. There was a large terminal building and several smaller buildings and hangers. It was just as described, abandoned. There wasn't a vehicle or person in sight.

"Well," said Cam, "it's mostly asphalt. Lots of weeds growing out of the cracks." He turned his head and gave his co-pilot a smirk.

Nigel returned a coy expression and shrugged his shoulders.

"Get your things and tighten your buckle."

"There you go again with that buckle business."

Cam made his approach. In the seconds before the wheels touched the ground, he unknowingly held his breath. His nerves didn't settle until the plane came to a complete stop. Then he exhaled. Surprisingly, the landing went much better than he expected.

Nigel played it off like it was nothing, but there was a side of him that had said a quiet little prayer. Not so much for their safety, but for the plane. It would have made him sick if anything wrong happened. "See. I told you," said Nigel. "Easy-shmeezy."

Cam said nothing and nodded as he taxied the plane to the deserted terminal.

"Kind of creepy looking, isn't it?" said Nigel.

The paint was badly faded and peeling from the building. Shards of glass littered the pavement. More windows were broken than not. An old, steel aircraft ladder once used to board and deboard passengers sat out in the open, covered in rust, surrendering to the elements. Between the terminal and the runway, a thin strip of shredded nylon flew in the air from atop a pole that once hosted a large windsock.

Cam looked around. "Yeah, I can't wait to get out of here. Come on. I'll get the door."

They stood outside the plane, shook hands, and raised their voices to speak over the engines.

"Thanks, Cam. I really appreciate it."

He nodded and smiled. "I'd say it was my pleasure, but..."

"Oh, stop being such a sourpuss. Now get out of here. I have a hike ahead of me. I'll call you when I'm settled."

"Be safe."

Nigel turned around, walked away, and yelled, "There you go again! Taking the fun out of everything."

Cam chuckled as he watched his friend cross the tarmac. Then he ducked back in the plane and closed the door.

Nigel found the gate locked, but he had his choice of holes in the fence to climb through. He stepped out on the street that ran along the airport. Placencia Road. He looked both ways. Not a car in sight. He threw his bag over his shoulder and headed east toward the shore, just a few miles away. Shortly after starting down the road, the sound of Cam taking off and climbing to the heavens interrupted his stride. He stopped to watch and wave. *Thanks again, buddy.*

About thirty minutes into his walk, he still hadn't seen another car. That all changed when a cranky old truck backfired behind him. Nigel turned and stopped. It approached, slowed, and stopped next to him. An old, well weathered-man sat behind the wheel. Sitting next to him was a boy. The truck was a flatbed, loaded down with bananas and a variety of citrus. The boy leaned out the window to look at the hiker. The old man reached across and pulled the boy out of the way. "Where are you going, son?"

With Belize being a former British colony, English is widely spoken along with Spanish, and to a lesser extent, Kriol or Belizean Creole. That made things easier.

"I'm just hiking the countryside, sir. On my way to Placencia."

"We are too!" said the boy.

"Hush up," said the old man, looking at the boy. "My grandson speaks out of turn. But he is right, we're headed that way to deliver fresh produce to some hotels. We have little room in the truck, but if you'd like a lift, jump on the back."

Nigel looked down the road in the direction he was going, then back the other way to gauge his progress. He looked at the old man and reached across to offer his hand. "Sounds great. Thanks."

The old man shook Nigel's hand and said, "Call me Pops and this is my grandson, Pablo."

"Just call me Chief."

They made several stops as they made their way down the coast. Nigel was more than willing to help offload and carry the bundles. It was the least he could do. He stayed with them until they finished the deliveries. The last stop was at the Placencia Beach Club. When he parted ways with Pops and Pablo, the old man refused to take a twenty-dollar bill. He waved it off. "Don't be silly. It was our pleasure, and thanks for your help."

Nigel waved and smiled as he watched Pops head down the road, grinding through the gears with the occasional backfire between shifts.

He turned to look around. First things first. He needed a car. He searched Google Maps and found Koool Car Rental. It was only a block away. He walked that way while he read the reviews. There were only seven. The place came in at 3.3 stars, but that was because of a single one-star review bitching about being scammed out of several thousands of dollars. Most other reviews were 5 stars. He stopped walking and stood in front of the office, trying to decide. Then a guy with a friendly smile came out and waved. *Huh! What did the Osmonds say? One bad apple don't spoil the whole bunch girl...* Nigel waved back and walked up to the guy. They shook hands.

"Looking for a car?" asked the guy.

"That seems to be the case. But I pay in cash."

"Oh, no credit card."

"I hate them."

"Well, come on in. I'll see what I can do."

"Great."

They went inside and the man went behind the counter. Nigel pulled a fan of hundred-dollar bills from his wallet. Then he put a driver's license on the counter.

The guy picked it up to study it. "So, Mr. Horton, how long do you need the car?"

Ten minutes later, Nigel left, driving a white Jeep Patriot, and the manager had cash in his pocket.

Second things second. Nourishment. He drove around and settled on the Pickled Parrot. For three reasons: it looked cool, the reviews were good, and more importantly, Dr. Benita's medical clinic was within walking distance. He had a cheeseburger and fries. They didn't have Diet Coke, so he settled for bottled water. It was all excellent, and he felt fueled up.

Seven and a half minutes later, he entered the medical clinic. The receptionist tilted her head with mild recognition. She spoke her brand of very broken English, but Nigel picked up on it. *Can I help you?*

Nigel pointed to his foot. "Stingray. I'm here to follow up with the doctor."

She nodded and held up a finger and left to get another woman with much better communication skills.

"Yes," she said. Then, "Oh, I remember you now. It's been some time ago." She rustled through some loose paperwork. "And the name?"

"Logan."

She kept looking, searched on the computer, and spoke to the screen. "Do you have an appointment?"

"No."

"Oh..."

Nigel slid the twenty-dollar bill refused by Pops across the counter. It was accepted. "But I will wait as long as I have to, if she can work me in."

"I'll see what I can do. Please take a seat."

He did, and she disappeared somewhere in the back.

There were three other people in the waiting room. Shortly after sitting down, a door opened and a nurse he remembered stood at the door and called one patient back. *What was her name? Maria. Yes, Maria.* She saw Nigel sitting and sent a smile his way as she escorted the patient in.

The clock on the wall showed a few minutes past two. He looked at his watch. It said 1507 Key West time. Patients came and went, and he now had waited for over two hours. It was just him and another waiting, and he was fine with it all. Without question, his time spent waiting would be the easiest part of the entire operation. And what the wait did was give him time to rehearse what and how he would approach the discussion. At a quarter past four, the other patient was called back. Maria looked at Nigel and said, "Sorry for the wait. She will see you next."

Nigel nodded. "No apology needed. I'm the one showing up unannounced."

With fifteen minutes left before closing, the last patient left, and Maria came out. "Mr. Logan. She will see you now."

Nigel got up and walked toward Maria. She noticed his walk to be fine, and that he suffered from no discomfort. "It seems you have healed nicely."

"I have. Thanks to you guys."

She led him back to the same examination room that he occupied the first time. "Have a seat and take off your shoe and sock."

She left, and he kept the shoe on. Five minutes later, Dr. Cabrera entered the room carrying his chart. This time she entered with a smile, and it made her even more beautiful than their first encounter. She saw his shoe was still on. She pulled out a chair and sat. "Maria said that you seem fine. Your shoe is still on, so obviously it doesn't need examining. What can I help you with?"

Nigel stood and walked over to a table as he spoke. "First to thank you and to show my appreciation for taking such good care of me." A box of tissues sat on the table. He grabbed it and went back to sit on the exam table. "And to help you."

"Help me?"

"Yes..."

She leaned forward and tilted her head, confused. "Why are you here? Help me with what?"

"Getting out of here."

She straightened up, stood, and turned away with a jerk.

"Listen, I'm not sure how to tell you this, so I'm just going to say it. I know what they did to your husband, Alejandro. And I know why you are here, and it certainly isn't because you love Belize and being away from your two children."

She turned around with a snap. "What do you know?"

"I know he loved you very much, and that he couldn't stand being away from you and the children. He was coming for you." He offered the box of tissues. She snatched a couple and wiped her eyes. "That's why he snuck out of Venezuela. He was going to collect the children, then come for you."

She said nothing.

"I'm here to help him finish what he started."

"That is impossible. And how do you know all this?"

"It's a long story, but just know I have Cuban friends with ears and eyes, in and outside of your homeland. These friends are prepared to help. One actually insists."

"What you are saying is nonsense. Even if you could get me out of this place, once they discover I'm gone, I'll never see my children again."

"Nope. What if I told you there was a plan to prevent that and get the children out as well?"

"What plan?"

"Well… to be honest. I'm not exactly sure. That is being developed now."

"Get out. I don't need to hear anymore. Leave now. Please."

Nigel stood. "I'm sorry. I didn't mean to upset you. But I won't give up. I'm kind of wired that way. I'll be back tomorrow. I feel a stomach virus coming on." He headed toward the door.

She turned to watch him leave. "Who are you?"

Nigel turned. "My name is in that chart you are holding. More importantly, I'm a friend of a friend who needs my help… to help you. I can be trusted. That's all you need to know."

"You need to leave."

"I will, but answer one question for me. It's been four years since you've seen your children. You are supposed to stay at least another year, and there is no way to know if your government will honor that. You are worth much more to them here than there. So, here is what I want to know. Forget the time you have left here. Do you really want to spend one more day away from Lucia and Antonio?"

"You! You know their names!"

Nigel said nothing, and she burst into tears.

"That's what I thought." He walked back to the tissue box and offered it. She took it.

"I'll see you tomorrow or the next day. Just know I'll be around. Maybe I'll make an appointment next time."

Chapter Twenty-Seven

Nigel waited and watched from the Jeep. Some of the other nurses and staff left and went to their vehicles, laughing and joking. Happy to be off work. Shortly thereafter, a white Chevy Impala sedan pulled up. Two men took up the front seat. Nigel looked at his watch. 1730. A single toot of the horn brought Dr. Cabrera and Maria out of the building. Maria locked up the clinic, and they both got in the back of the car. Nigel watched as the two men turned around to speak to their passengers. Then, as the car pulled away, Nigel fired up the Jeep.

He maintained a safe distance to follow as the Chevy made a few turns and ended up traveling north on Placencia Road. After a few miles, it made a right. When Nigel started his turn, he saw the sedan stopping at the very end of the street, so he pulled over and parked. He watched the doctor and Maria get out. Dr. Cabrera exchanged words with the two men, then followed Maria toward what looked to be a small apartment building. Nigel pretended to be looking at his phone as the Impala passed by. When the coast was clear, he eased down the road for a better look. They were staying at Palm Frond Suites. It looked small; four, maybe five suites, but it was on the water, facing the Caribbean Sea. It had that going for it.

Now that Nigel knew where she lived, it was time to find a place to stay. He lucked up and found a vacant room just a few blocks away at Brisa by the Sea. The accommodations were clean and luxurious. After dropping his bag in the room, he walked around the beautifully manicured grounds. The professionally maintained beach was just a few steps away from the gorgeous pool and tiki bar. Stool seventeen was open, so he climbed aboard. A dark and beautiful bartender approached. She carried a million-dollar smile with teeth brighter and whiter than anything he could remember. Her hair was pulled tight in a ponytail and her dark brown eyes matched her soft, smooth skin. A gentle breeze came off the water and brought her scent to him before she arrived. *Damn*. When she was close enough, he read her name tag. "Shanda. Are all the women in Belize as beautiful as you?"

She smiled and winked. "No." She let that sink. "They are much prettier!"

"You are too humble."

She took a rag and cleaned a spot in front of him. "Thank you and welcome to Placencia. What may I get for you?"

"Diet Coke would be fine."

"Just a Diet Coke, no coconut or regular rum with it? Or how about some other tropical drink?"

"Thank you, but no. Maybe later."

"Coming up."

As she stepped away, Nigel pulled out his cell phone. Time to find out if these international calling plans work. He scrolled through his contacts and hit the dial button. After a while it started ringing, so maybe it was working.

Shortly after, Cam's voice answered. "So, you made it?"

"Yeah. Caught a ride on a banana truck." The bartender brought his drink, and he mouthed a *Thank You* to her. "It was like something from a movie. Stacks of bananas and boxes of oranges and grapefruit surrounded me as we bounced down the road. It was all good. I'm settled now, and dang this place is nice. How is Belize City?"

"Change of plans. Landed in Dangriga. It's on the water and closer to where you are. Much better than the big city. Got a room close to the airport and on the water. On the patio now, finishing up a little dinner. Food is good."

"Well, it's hard to complain about that."

"I have one. Complaint that is. They don't have any Wild Turkey, so I'm stuck, settling for your Jim Beam."

"Hey! Don't go hating on J.B. We aren't as acquainted as we once were, but I still consider him a friend."

"Whatever. Where did you end up?"

"A nice place on the water. Just a few blocks down the beach from where the doctor lives."

Knowing Cam didn't need or want any explicit details, Nigel gave him a watered-down version of his meeting with the doctor and how he followed her to her suite.

"So, yeah," said Nigel, "I'm positioned pretty well. And it is nothing short of amazing what less than a hundred and fifty bucks will get you in Placencia. A comparable place in Key West this time of year would easily fetch six to seven hundred a night, or maybe more."

"I'm paying closer to two hundred a night. And yeah, it is a value, but let me remind you... we are not on vacation."

"I know. I know, but I could get used to this." He waved to his bartender, and she approached. "Hold on, Cam." He held the phone so Cam could hear. "Shanda. By chance, do you have any Wild Turkey?"

"We do."

"Would you bring me one?"

Nigel smiled and brought the phone up to his ear. "Anyway, Cam. I'll let you go now. I'll be in touch soon."

Cam said nothing. Nigel looked at his screen. The call had ended. Two seconds later, his phone bonged with a text message. It was from Cam. Nigel read the terse message and laughed. *I hate you.*

Basilio, Javiero, and Riel watched as Fredrico stumbled away from the table and down the street.

"He seems to have some regrets. Perhaps shouldering some guilt," said Javiero.

"Regret. Guilt." said Basilio, "I don't care about any of that. Being loyal is one thing, but to betray your own people, your own family, that is a crime against humanity, unforgivable in my eyes."

Riel noticed a couple of fellas approaching the table, looking for a game. He held up a hand and pushed away from the table. "Here, grab another team. We are done. It's yours."

The three of them maintained a safe distance as they followed Fredrico down the street.

"So would someone explain to me what is going on?" asked Riel.

"My real name is Basilio Valdez. I am from Miami, and here to help Alejandro finish what he started. To export and unite what is left of his family and take them to a better life."

"And how do you expect to do that?"

"With Fredrico's assistance, I hope. It would be in his best interest."

"Good luck with that. Have you spoken with Dr. Benita about this?"

"I have a capable man on the ground in Placencia now, coordinating the effort. I should hear from him soon."

"What if she doesn't want to take the chance?"

"I'll do what I can to convince her, but if she still resists... I will have to let it go. It only works if she is willing."

"You make it sound like you have done this before?"

Basilio smiled. "It's what I do. Mostly with skilled cooks and chefs. They are in great demand back in the States."

Riel stopped. "Chefs?"

Javiero said, "Yeah... really?"

"Ha! Do either of you remember? It was several years back. Raul Castro's private chef went missing."

"Ahhh... Yes," said Riel. "I remember that. MININT was on full alert. They scoured the country looking for him."

Javiero was amazed. "That was you?"

"I don't do it alone. I can't do it alone. I have help."

"You. You smuggled them out?" said Riel.

"Oh! I hate that word. It sounds so, so wrong and illegal. No, I export chefs to a better life. Before Raul and his punks knew what happened, the chef and his wife were in Mexico, heading to the U.S. border."

A painful cry sounded ahead of them, and they turned to see Fredrico face down in the gutter.

They started that way, but Basilio put his hands out to stop Riel and Javiero. "Please let me, help him."

Basilio ran to Fredrico, who had trouble getting to his feet. He got a good hold under his arm and lifted him up. "There you go, old man. Steady up. Can you make it?"

Fredrico looked at Basilio. "Who... who are you?"

"It is me. Juan. Remember? We were just playing dominos. I'm afraid I did you no favors by bringing that last bottle of rum. Where are you going?"

"Mi casa."

"Then let me help you home."

Fredrico straightened up and looked back in the direction he had come. Javiero and Riel were standing there in the distance. "Those bastards don't know what they are talking about."

Basilio looked back at them, too. "I am quite sure you are right. But forget about all that disturbing talk. A disloyal man is dead. Let's get you home."

Fredrico nodded.

"Show me the way."

The house was only a few blocks further on the outskirts of town. Twice Basilio had to catch Fredrico from falling down in the street.

Once inside, Basilio looked around the small room and found an easy chair. "Let's get you sitting down, old man."

Again, Fredrico nodded. Once settled, Fredrico looked at the stranger and said, "Gracias."

"De nada."

Fredrico closed his eyes.

"Lo lamento, my friend. I am sorry we upset you so much at the game. I know nothing of what they say."

Fredrico slowly shook his head from side to side and said nothing.

Basilio looked around the room and found evidence of children everywhere. "I guess the kids are in school. How many?"

The old man squinted to look. "Dos. My grandchildren."

"And their madre?"

Basilio watched as the old man's lips quivered and a tear fell from an eye. "Working... The children miss her so much."

"Where is she?"

Fredrico's eyes opened wider, and he looked upon Basilio with great suspicion. "And who did you say you were? Do you know my Benita?"

"Nope. Just wanting to help."

Fredrico feigned a more sobering look. "Thanks for getting me home, but I need no more of your help. I think you should leave."

Before shutting the door, Basilio gave the old man one last look. His eyes were closed, and his head hung back. Slowly, at first, his head drooped forward until it bounced with a snap. He was out cold. *Pathetic old man*, he thought. *To hell with you and your kind. I'll be back when you least expect it, and you probably won't like it.* He gave the door a little slam and Fredrico's eyes fluttered, but only for a second or two.

Out by the street, he paused. Something caught his eye, and he looked to his right. Then he looked back the way he came, and, instead of heading back toward town, he took a right and headed out of town. From there, it quickly became rural and agricultural, except for the cemetery less than a quarter of a mile away.

This is where the bastards killed them. He walked around, looking at the headstones and crypts. He was maybe in there for seven minutes when he stopped in his tracks. Two messy and unclean headstones still had splattered blood, brain, and skull remnants. Blood that had oxidized in the air and had now turned a dark brown, almost black. *They didn't even clean it up.* He turned around and headed to town. P*erhaps I won't either.*

Back at the Park he met up with Javiero. Riel had gone back to the shop.

"Well?" inquired Javiero.

"Well, I've seen enough. It all makes me sick. Let's go back to Carlito's."

Chapter Twenty-Eight

Early the next morning, Nigel sat in his Jeep down the street from the doctor's apartment building. He patiently observed the comings and goings from the side and rear-view mirrors. At 0740 and halfway through his second large cup of coffee, two things happened. First, he saw the white Impala turn onto the road. Inside were the same two guys from the afternoon before. This time, he got a better look. The second thing to happen was a sudden need to bleed his bladder. *Crap! Perfect timing, Logan*. It hadn't built to a critical stage yet, but the large caffeine loading could quickly change that.

He watched the car stop and blow its horn three times. Dr. Benita and Maria exited the same unit and hurried to the car. The clinic opened at eight and was just a few blocks away, but maybe they felt they were running late. Once the Impala hung a left on Placencia Road to head south, Nigel started the car and put it in drive. He followed them to the clinic. That part of the tail would be obvious, but he wanted to find out where these guys were coming from. He parked around the corner and waited. His knees bounced in and out. A couple minutes later, his fingers drummed on the steering wheel and kept perfect time with his knees. "Come on, dammit. Get out of there," he said to the windshield.

Moments later, the Impala emerged, and he followed them back to Placencia Road, where they went north. And in no big hurry at all. He spoke to the guys in the Impala. "Go, dammit. Go." Then he spoke to himself. "Don't, go. Don't go. Don't go."

Nigel made a mental note of a small place on the right. Carmen's Kitchen. It was a roadside eatery, very local, and put together as a hodge-podge shack with mostly open-air dining, colorful picnic tables, and an inside area. Nigel mentally prayed for a bathroom.

A few blocks later, the brake lights of the Impala glowed, and a left turn signal was added. It turned in. Nigel drove by and gave it a quick look. It seemed to be a government building of sorts. He could study it later, after a quick stop at Carmen's. As he braked and turned the car around, he cheered himself on. "No! No! No! Don't go, dammit! NOT NOW! DON'T GOOOO!"

Carmen, the staff, and the other patrons, an obvious mix of locals and tourists, were laughing as he emerged from the single restroom. Lucky for him and Carmen, it had recently been vacated. If he had been forced to dance around and wait for somebody to come out, it would have certainly meant a disaster. He noticed that most of the restaurant's eyes were on him, which would have embarrassed most folks, but Nigel wiped the real sweat from his brow and said, "That was a close one!"

After a few chuckles, people went back to their breakfast and Nigel grabbed stool seventeen at the makeshift bar that stretched across a long window.

A skinny dark man, wearing a sweat-stained bandana on his head, a Jimmy Buffett Parrot Head t shirt, and an apron once bleached white, asked in a thick Jamaican accent, "What can I get for you, mon?"

"Not coffee. I've had my fill." The menu was limited and hung on the wall. He pointed. "I'll take the Full Breakfast."

"All da way?"

"Yes, whatever that means, and a Diet Coke."

"Gotcha!"

Nigel turned around to take in his surroundings. He was no longer the center of attention. He was thankful for that. After a few minutes, he heard, "Da Diet Coke."

Nigel spun around and grabbed the glass. "Thank you. What is your name?"

"Domingo, but de call me Jimmy, cause I love da mistah Buffett. What is your name?"

Nigel stuck out his hand. "I'm Jimmy too. Last name, Horton. Jim Horton from Sanibel Island."

Jimmy scratched his head in thought.

"Sanibel," said Nigel. "It's a barrier island west of Fort Myers, Florida."

"Neva been."

"It is a beautiful place, but I'd have to say Placencia and Belize have it beat."

"Ya. Tis nice, huh, mon?"

Jimmy then looked over Nigel's shoulders and said, "Sam! Bernard! Wah Gwaan! Da usual?"

Nigel took a sip of his DC and heard someone say, "Si."

As he turned around, he almost inhaled his soda. It was Dr. Benita's chauffeur and sidekick. They walked up and took the empty stools next to him. The one next to Nigel nodded to acknowledge him. Nigel nodded back and said, "Good morning."

They both were cheerful enough when they replied with the same.

"So," started Jimmy, "did yuh geet da sweet doctor ta work dis morning?"

"Yeah," said one of them, "and it's getting old. She isn't going anywhere, but suddenly the damn Cubans insist we see that she gets to work and home. It's crazy."

"Why?" asked Jimmy.

"Don't know. Here lately it's like they are worried she will take off. Yesenia, the office manager, is supposed to call us if she leaves during the day. It is all stupid."

"I hope she doesn't leave. She is a damn good doctor." Jimmy lifted a finger. "She stitched me up good last week when I almost cut off dis finger."

Nigel looked at the cut and immediately thought, *Shouldn't you be wearing a glove while working?*

"I know," said the guy next to Nigel. "She is the best doctor we've had in years."

The other guy said, "Not to mention pretty and sweet."

Nigel jumped into the conversation. "Are you guys talking about the doctor at the clinic? Oh, hell... what's her name? Cabbri... Cabo..."

"Cabrera," said Jimmy.

"Yes!" Nigel slapped the bar. "She is outstanding. I showed up there a while back with a massive stingray barb shoved up my foot. She had to cut it out. She was incredible."

"Dat be her," said Jimmy.

Nigel focused on the other two. "I didn't mean to eavesdrop," he lied, "but you say you have to escort her around?" Nigel reached out to shake the first guy's hand. "I'm sorry. I'm Jim, but not like your Mr. Buffett over here." Nigel slid Sam a business card. "I'm just Jim. Jim Horton. Boring I know."

The first guy chuckled. "I'm Sam and this is Bernard."

Bernard gave a little salute.

Sam continued, "We're detectives for the city and police station. And yeah. Dr. Cabrera is Cuban, and all of a sudden, the embassy in Belize City wants us on a babysitting mission. She and Maria normally walk to work. It is crazy."

Jimmy laughed from behind the window. "Yes, how do yuh say it? From dat movie? I remember now. Sam and Bernard are driving Ms. Daisy! Ha!"

"Shut up, Domingo," said Bernard.

"Why would they want you to do that? Keep tabs on her?" asked Nigel.

"Because they are bastards," said Sam.

"I take it you don't like them much," said Nigel.

"The Cubans from the embassy are pushy and bossy," said Sam. "They run around giving orders. Like this is their country. Dr. Cabrera... She is different. We like her. The others can go to hell for all I care."

Jimmy served up the breakfast through the window. The full breakfast comprised eggs, beans, cheese, ham, and a flour tortilla. It was good, and everyone ate in silence. Not another word was mentioned about Dr. Benita.

Nigel hopped off the bar, paid for all three breakfasts and tipped Jimmy well. As he left, he couldn't help but think, *Almost pissing yourself can be a good thing*.

Nigel sat in his Jeep outside the clinic for about an hour. He contemplated keeping his promise and going back in to talk to her, but decided against it. And just sitting there did nothing to move the ball down the field, so he drove back to his room to get the sat phone. Needing a clear view of the sky and wanting privacy, he walked down to the beach to walk along the surf. Basilio answered in four rings.

"Nigel! My friend. How are things going?"

"Just dandy. And you?"

"We are in position. Just waiting to hear what you have learned."

"Dr. Cabrera is fine and healthy. I spoke with her yesterday afternoon and explained why I was back in town. I can tell she is scared and doesn't want to lose her children. Local authorities escort her to and from work at the direction of your embassy in Belize City."

"It is not my embassy, my friend. So, those escorting her are working closely with the thugs. Is that what you are saying?"

"Not exactly. They like and respect the good doctor."

Nigel explained what he had garnered from Sam and Bernard and the contempt they felt for the Cuban officials.

"So, my friend, what you are saying is these two men could be assets and not necessarily a liability?"

"I don't know, Basilio. I've only met and bought their breakfast once. But what we can bank on is they like Dr. Cabrera a lot more than the Cuban authorities. What have you found out?"

"The doctor's father is a weasel, and he still has the children. By all appearances and from reports, they are being taken care of, but they miss their mother."

"So, what's next?"

"You need to talk with her again. Find out if she wants out and to be united with her children. If she does, things will move quickly."

"If I had to guess, it would be tough for me to convince her, even if she wants to. She has no reason to trust me. This has all been so sudden to her."

The line went quiet for a while. For a second, Nigel thought they had dropped a satellite. "Basilio... Are you there?"

"Yes, my friend. I am thinking."

"Of?"

"I am thinking I need to press the issue. Move faster than I earlier planned. And if things don't work out, both you and I will need to find our way back home as soon as possible."

"I'm not sure I like the sound of that."

"Well, I'm afraid you might be right. She will need additional motivation to convince her. Will you see her later? After she gets off work, maybe?"

"I can try."

"No trying, my friend. Find her, Nigel Logan. Talk to her. Then call me sometime after seven Miami time. I will talk with her. If she refuses, we run like hell."

Chapter Twenty-Nine

Instead of sitting and waiting in the Jeep. Nigel took a chance by pacing the sidewalk up and down Dr. Cabrera's street. He was walking toward the car when the Impala made its turn. Nigel ignored the car and the people inside, but at six-three, two hundred thirty pounds, there was no way they could ignore his presence.

Inside the car, Dr. Cabrera and Maria noticed him first, then looked at each other with surprise. Then Bernard said, "Hey, Sam. There's that Horton fella we met this morning."

Benita and Maria looked at each other again. Benita leaned forward. "Y'all know him?"

"Know him? No. We met him at Carmen's this morning. Nice guy. He bought our breakfast."

Bernard turned to look at her. "You should know him, too. He said you extracted one hell of a stingray barb out of his foot."

Not knowing what to say, Dr. Cabrera said, "I thought he looked familiar. What did you say his name was again?"

Sam stopped the car in front of the apartment, and Bernard said, "Horton." Then he looked at Sam.

Sam looked at Bernard and said, "Jim."

Then, together, they said, "Jim Horton."

Benita flopped back in her seat and looked at Maria. They were thinking the same thing. That's not his real name. Then the doctor said, "Yeah, now I remember. Don't you Maria? Jim Horton. Nasty stingray barb."

"Is that the one that came in self-medicated on Big Titty Rum?" asked Maria.

"That's the one."

All four laughed and turned to look.

Nigel kept walking. Just out for a little casual stroll. When he got to the end of the street, Dr. Cabrera and Maria watched Nigel Logan turn left and keep walking. Sam and Bernard watched Jim Horton do the same.

Inside the apartment, Dr. Cabrera prepared dinner. Ceviche with black beans and rice. Little was said during the meal. Distractions and concerns flooded Benita's mental space, and Maria had questions bouncing around in her head. Once dinner was over and the kitchen and dishes cleaned up, Maria couldn't stand it any longer. "What is going on, Benita? There is something you are not telling me. I can see it on your face."

"It's nothing."

"Yes. It is something. What? Who is he?"

"His real name is Nigel Logan. I think. That was on his ID."

"Then why would he tell Sam and Bernard his name was Jim Horton?"

"I can't be sure."

"But you have an idea, right?"

Dr. Cabrera went quiet.

"Benitaaaaa?"

"Okay. Okay. Remember when he came in yesterday?"

"For the follow-up? The one he clearly didn't need."

"Exactly. Well... It's all so disturbing."

"What? Tell me."

"He knows everything about Alejandro. He knows MININT had him killed, and he knows why I am here, and you too, I guess. Even knows the names of my children! He says he wants to help me get out of here and away from the medical brigade."

"If you do that, you'll never see Lucia and Antonio again."

"I know, but he said people were prepared to get them out of Cuba, so we could all be together again."

Maria rubbed her head and walked over to the big picture window that overlooked the Caribbean Sea. "That sounds crazy."

"I know. And he said he wasn't going away."

"Benita?"

"He said that he couldn't give up."

"Benita?"

"He said that..."

"Benita! He isn't going away, and he isn't giving up. Come here."

Dr. Cabrera joined Maria at the window. She looked down at the beach and found Nigel looking up at them from behind a couple of Adirondack chairs nestled in the sand. After a few awkward moments, Nigel gave a friendly wave.

"Oh dear," said the doctor.

Then they watched Nigel take a seat in one of the chairs.

"What are you going to do, Benita?"

The doctor held her head. "I don't know. Go talk to him, I guess. He seems harmless enough."

"Harmless and dangerous at the same time."

"Dangerous... maybe, but not to me... I think. I'll be right back."

From behind him, he heard the shifting kicks of sand and quiet footsteps. Then they stopped. "So, which is it? Logan or Horton?"

Nigel turned to see her standing in the light of the early dusk. She no longer wore her medical scrubs. Her feet were bare. She wore tight, faded blue jeans with the knees worn through, and an untucked, oversized, white short-sleeved blouse. Her dark hair was pulled back into a ponytail. She was stunning. The attraction made it difficult for Nigel to remember that she had just lost her loving husband.

"It's Logan, and it wouldn't do me any good to lie to you. It is your trust and confidence I need to earn."

"May I sit down?"

"You would disappoint me if you didn't."

The doctor looked up at the window. Maria stood there, keeping a close eye on any strange developments. Benita blew Maria a sweet little kiss, then sat down.

They were quiet for a while, then Nigel said, "I'm sorry about yesterday. I didn't mean to or want to upset you. It wasn't my desire."

"What do you desire?"

"Like I said yesterday, to help you."

"What if I don't want your help? I mean, yes. I hate being away from my sweet children. Four years is a long time to be away from them. Aside from losing my Alejandro..." She paused and pushed away the uncontrollable tears that flooded her eyes. "Not having my children is the worst part of my nightmare. While I detest the circumstances, I could have it much worse. I could serve in some third-world dump with little to no resources. Here, the people are kind and appreciate the care that Maria and I provide."

"Maria, your nurse? She too is part of the brigade?"

"Yes."

Nigel turned to look up at the window. Maria beamed down at them. Then he turned to look at the doctor. "And I gather she is also a good friend?"

"The best."

"Does she have family and children left behind too?"

"No, her parents died two years ago from influenza, and she has no children. While the loss of her parents is tragic and painful, she is lucky, very lucky. She loves it here. If I had to guess, when the time comes to return to Cuba, she will somehow disappear. For her sake, I hope she is successful."

"What about your sake? Do you want to return home?"

"Now, I'm afraid it is no longer my home. Only Cuba, but if that is where I have to go to be with my children, so be it."

"But if you are with them somewhere else, would you take that chance?"

"I don't know. Probably not."

Nigel looked at his watch. It was 1913, so he pulled out and powered up the satellite phone.

CHAPTER THIRTY

Earlier that afternoon, Basilio went back to the park to find Fredrico. He was there, as predicted. Riel was with him as they sat on a bench, waiting to challenge a nearby table. Basilio approached them.

"Riel. Fredrico. Buenas tardes."

Riel smiled and nodded. Fredrico didn't and said nothing.

"Fredrico? Are we feeling better today?"

"Si. But no thanks to you."

Basilio burst out in laughter and held up his hands. "Guilty! I am so sorry. Perhaps I can make it up to you later."

"I don't think so."

Basilio's jovial deportment took on a more somber note as he said, "Well, I feel I would be negligent in my duties if I didn't try."

Fredrico said nothing.

"Señors," said Basilio with a bow of his head, "I bid you farewell. Have a grand match. I wish you both fabulous success."

Riel and Fredrico watched Basilio walk away.

"I don't know about him," said Fredrico.

"How do you mean? He seems okay. Javiero seems to like and trust him."

"I don't know. There is something about the way he acts. Like he's not... not... Cuban."

"Oh, Fredrico, what are you talking about? That is nonsense. How do you think he acts?"

Fredrico looked at Riel. "American. I've seen how the U.S. tourists in Cienfuegos act and carry themselves."

"Fredrico, you don't know what you are talking about. Now come on, we're up. Grab that bottle."

Basilio walked down the sidewalk less than three blocks. He knew where he was going and finally stopped at a chain-link fence. Behind it was the playground for Manuel Santiago Elementary School. Children joyfully ran around and played. Some on swings, some on the slides, some running and kicking after a football that got bounced about. Basilio wondered if any of the children belonged to Dr. Cabrera. He figured he'd find out soon enough.

Riel and Fredrico played dominos until a little after four in the afternoon. Yes, there had been plenty of rum. Fredrico got a healthy shine about himself, but nothing like the day before. He excused himself from the table in order to be home when the children arrived from school.

Basilio waited just inside an alley where he could see the road that led to the house. Once he saw Fredrico ease by, Basilio fell in behind, keeping a safe distance. Fredrico went inside his house and Basilio found a bench at a bus stop, a few houses down, to rest, wait, and watch. About forty minutes later, he noticed a little boy coming down the street, holding the hand of an older girl. Ah, he thought, *this must be Lucia and Antonio*. Lucia looked to be in her early teens and Antonio was much younger. They were beautiful and happy children, too young to know that a much better life existed beyond the island. A life that soon awaited them, or at least he hoped that would be the case. Once they were safely inside, he got up and walked back into town for an early dinner. Then he would return to put things into motion.

Fredrico sat in his favorite chair, listening to the radio as he sipped rum. Antonio played with the only toy he had, loading a string around an old wooden top that would again be slung to spin on the floor. Lucia sat at the kitchen table, finishing up her homework. It was a normal evening in the small town of Palmira until a loud knock came from the front door. It startled all three of them. Visitors were rare.

Fredrico turned off the radio and answered the door.

Three men dressed in green MININT uniforms brushed by Fredrico as they entered uninvited. Lucia quickly ran to her brother to hold him and ease his fears.

"What is the meaning of this?" Fredrico demanded.

One man said, "Sit. Somebody wants to talk to you."

"I will do no such thing. Get out of my house. You have no business with me."

Moments later, Basilio entered the house. "You are right, Fredrico. They have no business with you. I do."

"What is this all about?"

"Confessions. I'll confess my sins, if you'll confess yours."

Basilio moved in close so he could speak without the children hearing. He strongly doubted the children knew what role their grandfather played in their father's death, and for their sake, he wanted to keep it that way. "Alejandro, my friend. Alejandro."

"You are no friend of mine. Who are you? And don't say Juan."

Basilio backed away. "My name is Basilio Valdez. I am a friend of your daughter, Benita. I am here to help her, the children, and you, if you are smart."

Another of the green soldiers looked at his watch, then interrupted. "Basilio. It is a little after seven. It is about time."

"Very good. Go outside and wait for it."

"What are you talking about, and what does the ministry have to do with it?"

Basilio looked at the soldiers. "Ah, I couldn't do what I do without them."

"Which is?"

"Help my Cuban brothers and sisters find a new and wonderful life away from this godforsaken country. I'm here to help your daughter and the children. And like I said, if you are smart, you will follow along. You have no idea what pleasures of life you are missing."

Basilio walked over to the children.

"Leave them alone!" demanded Fredrico.

Basilio stopped and turned around. "Please, Fredrico. There is no reason to yell. You are scaring the little ones." Then Basilio turned and sat on the floor to face the kids. "Please do not be afraid. There is nothing to be scared of." He looked at the girl first. "So, you must be Lucia."

She nodded her head.

Basilio added a little wink and a white lie. "Your mother was right. She told me you were beautiful."

Lucia smiled. "You know our madre?"

"Yes, oddly. I know all the hearts and minds of those who seek a better life. So yes, I know your mother well."

"Who are you?" she asked.

"I'm like an uncle you've never met. Call me Uncle Basilio."

From over Basilio's shoulder, came. "He's not your uncle, Lucia."

Basilio never took his eyes off her. "That's enough, Fredrico. You are confusing the children." Then he focused on the boy. He puffed out his chest and spoke in a playful, deep voice. "And you must be Antonio. You aren't scared, are you?"

He shook his head.

"That's what I thought. You are a brave one."

"I'm a brave one too," confirmed Lucia.

"Well, of course, I already knew that. I have a little question for the two of you. How would you like to go on a little trip with your Uncle Basilio?"

"That is enough!" Fredrico yelled. "The children are not going anywhere. Now get out of my house."

Basilio smiled at the children. They looked confused. "Everything is going to be alright. I need to speak to your grandfather."

He calmly rose and walked over to Fredrico. "Here is what is going to happen. We will leave soon. Very soon. The children will go with us. It is entirely up to you, but I insist you go as well. You will not regret it, and doing so will make things much easier. Plus, it might help keep the children calm."

"The children are staying here!"

"Whether the children stay or leave isn't up to you."

"What are you talking about?"

There was a knock at the door. One of the MININT soldiers answered it, took a message, and came back in to make an announcement. "Basilio. They are on the line."

A huge smile stretched across Basilio's face. He looked at his watch. It was a quarter after seven. "Fredrico. I will be right back." As he left to go outside, he told the two remaining soldiers, "Keep an eye on him. Don't let him do anything stupid."

Basilio took the phone. "Nigel, my good man. How are things?"

"I'm enjoying a pleasant evening on the beach with Dr. Cabrera. We are getting to know..." He turned to make eye contact with her. "... and trust one another. How are things with you?"

"That will depend on the next few minutes, but if I had to guess, I'd say splendid. Please, give the phone to the good doctor."

Nigel reached over and offered the phone. "Here. He would like to talk to you."

"Who is it?"

"That special friend of yours wanting to help. A guy who can be trusted. A guy that makes things happen. I'm not exactly sure what he has in mind, but he wishes to speak with you."

She took the phone. Her only word in English to Basilio was *hello*. After she listened for a while, the conversation went into a rapid exchange of Spanish. Basilio must have mentioned Nigel, because Dr. Cabrera turned to look at him, smiling. Suddenly, she gave a violent gasp and covered her mouth. Tears exploded from her eyes, and she made no attempt to wipe them. She shook all over, covered the mouthpiece, and looked at Nigel. "He is with my father and children. He's gone to get them, so I can speak with them."

Moments later, Nigel watched as her face glowed as she spoke with her children. Never before had he heard such excited crying and laughter. It was a pure, joyous, Latin expression of love, devotion, and regret.

When she was done with them, her deportment shifted and Nigel caught her words, hearing her say *Papa*. The conversation was loving and sad at the same time. It was a mix of anger, frustration, and compassion. There was no doubt they were speaking of Alejandro. When they were done talking, she looked at Nigel, and he reached over and used his thumbs to push away her tears. Then she went back to talking. Nigel was pretty sure Basilio was back on the line. She did a lot of listening. There was some head nodding, and he caught the occasional *Si. Si*. She seemed agreeable. Then, after a brief pause, she started talking again. This time, to Lucia, the passionate reunion talk was over. Mother was now giving direct instruction and encouragement. When she was done, she sniffled, smiled, handed the phone back to Nigel, and said, "Why are you doing this?"

"Because it's the right thing to do. Plus, after witnessing what just happened, there is no doubt in my mind that I'm here for all the right reasons."

Nigel put the phone to his ear. "Basilio, where are we?"

"We are on the move, my friend. So are you and the doctor. Let her collect her things and get her out of there. Take her somewhere safe. Things will happen very fast, so move quickly. Keep the phone charged. I will call you in the morning."

Chapter Thirty-One

Maria watched as Nigel and her friend got out of the Adirondacks and hugged. She could tell Benita was crying, and by the time the two of them came in the front door, Maria stood just inside to greet them. "What is going on, Benita?"

The doctor ran to her nurse and friend. They embraced in the hall. "I spoke with my children."

"Lucia and Antonio?"

"Yes. On the phone. Lucia was so thrilled."

"What about Antonio?"

Benita broke down, held her open mouth with both hands and cried.

"Benita?"

She nodded her head and held up a finger. *Give me a second.* When she finished collecting herself, she said, "He sounded so grown, but he remembers only so much of me. He was barely four when we left. Lucia has done her best to keep my memory alive."

Maria said nothing, and Nigel stood quietly in the corner.

"THOSE BASTARDS! They took my motherhood away from me. My son! He barely remembers who I am. I'll never forgive them for that."

Maria took her friend into her arms, and they hugged. Maria consoled Benita, swinging her from side to side. She looked over her friend's shoulder to see a concerned Nigel waiting.

He said, "Dr. Cabrera... we need to get moving."

Maria broke the embrace so she and Benita could look at one another. "Get moving? What is going on?"

"I am leaving this place. To be with my children."

"But where?"

Dr. Cabrera turned to look at Nigel and said, "We're not exactly sure yet. The man in Cuba said it is probably best that way."

"What man?"

"The man bringing my children. His name is Basilio Valdez."

"I don't know, Benita. This all sounds so risky."

"I don't want to wait another year before I can see my children. And Mr. Logan is right..."

"Ah, excuse me," Nigel interrupted, "I'm no mister. How many times do I have to tell people? Please, call me Chief."

Dr. Cabrera ignored him. "... there is no guarantee they will let me go home. And if they do, who knows where else they might send me once I get back? No... I'm not willing to risk that."

Nigel stepped forward. "Maria. You are welcome to come too. You don't have to stay here either."

Maria kissed Benita on the cheek and walked away, stopping a few feet away. "No. I will stay." She turned around. "I love it here."

Nigel looked at the doctor, and she said, "Told you."

"Very well," said Nigel. "Your mind is made up, and we don't have a lot of time to change it."

Nigel waited by the front door.

Maria watched Benita pack what few things she needed. "I'm going to miss you."

Benita looked up from her small bag and zipped it up. "I'm going to miss you, too."

They walked arm in arm to where Nigel waited. "Are you ready?" he said.

The doctor took a deep breath. "No... but yes."

Nigel took her bag, and she turned to hug Maria one last time.

"What should I tell them?"

The doctor thought about it. "Tell them anything you want. The truth. I don't care."

Maria looked at Nigel. "Hey," he said, "I'm big on honesty, but there is no need to tell the truth, the whole truth, and nothing but the truth, so help you, God."

Maria's face contorted.

"What? Don't you ever watch Perry Mason or Matlock?"

She shook her head.

"Forget it. Tell them she left sometime in the night, and you don't know where she is. Cooperate with them. If you don't, they will suspect you. As a matter of fact, call and report her missing when you wake up. That way, you'll look even more innocent."

Dr. Cabrera reached for the door and opened it. "Let's go."

Nigel reached out and held Maria's hand. "Last chance."

She shook her head with a smile.

"Good luck then." And they slipped out the door.

Inside the Jeep, the doctor said, "I guess I now know how Alejandro felt when he fled."

"It's called... bravery."

She smiled. "Please, take me to the clinic. I have a couple of things I need to collect."

"I don't think that is such a good idea. What if someone sees you?"

"Please."

Nigel parked around the corner and left the engine running. "Please, be quick about it."

He watched her disappear, and he looked at his watch. 2245. Quarter to nine. The minutes of waiting seemed like hours. He looked around. There was little foot traffic. In the rearview, he saw a man walking toward the car. A dog led the way. As he passed in front of the car, Dr. Cabrera came around the corner. She stopped to talk to the man. *Crap! They know each other.* They spent way too much time speaking to each other, and they finally hugged before he continued on. She got in the car with another bag, and Nigel put them back in motion before she could buckle up.

"That is exactly why I didn't want to come here. Now someone has seen you out."

"Relax, Mr. Logan. Mr. Martinez is an old, sweet patient. He has an appointment next week. I didn't have the heart to tell him I wouldn't be there." She paused for a bit as Nigel turned north on Placencia Road.

"And this is why I needed to go back there."

From her bag, she pulled four pictures. Nigel glanced over as he drove. One was of a handsome man wearing surgical scrubs. He was arm and arm with Benita. Alejandro, no doubt. Another picture was of a young girl. Sweet smile and all the future good looks of her mother. Lucia. The third was of a tiny toddler. He was cute, sitting on a swing with his sister behind him. The fourth was a complete ensemble, all four of them together at the beach. "So, you see. I couldn't leave them behind."

"Yes, I do."

"Where are we going?"

"Have you ever been to Dangriga?"

She shook her head.

"Me either."

They were all gathered, standing out front. Basilio handed the phone back to one of the guys. "So, Fredrico. What is it going to be? Are you going to do the smart thing and come with the children?"

Fredrico glanced at the car sitting under the streetlight. "The children are going nowhere!"

Basilio looked at one of the green suits. "Please, take the children inside and pack a small travel bag."

When they were inside, Basilio looked at Fredrico. "You don't seem to understand. Their mother wants them to go, so they are going. She wants to see them. You should want to see her too, because you never will... once we are gone."

"You are going to take away what remains of my family. I will not stand for it."

"Just like you had Alejandro taken from Benita. Big difference though. This time, nobody she cares about is going to die."

"You don't understand. I never meant for that to happen."

"Yet, it did."

Fredrico looked at the ground and said nothing.

"So, I will ask you one last time, because time is something I don't have the luxury of. Are you coming or not?"

He said nothing.

Basilio grabbed him by the shoulder, swung him around, and pushed him toward the door. "You are an old fool. Get back in the house, sit in your chair, drink your rum, and stay out of the way."

A few minutes later, the children and men in green came out of the children's room. "Basilio, we are ready to go."

Lucia went to her grandpapa. "Where is your bag? We are going to see mama. Why are you crying?"

Fredrico looked upon his granddaughter and said, "I am not going. Here is where I belong."

Antonio ran to his sister's side. "No, grandpapa. You must come. Mama wants to see you too."

Lucia looked at Basilio. "We cannot leave him. He must go."

"But, sweetheart, he has decided," said Basilio. "And it is time to go. We must leave. Your Mama is waiting for you."

The children cried as they hugged their grandpapa one last time. Then Fredrico watched as they disappeared out the door with the green men.

Basilio walked over to him and said, "You know I can't leave you like this. Free to call and inform MININT. I have to tie you up. Trust me, though. It is only for tonight; somebody will come in the morning. I guarantee it."

Chapter Thirty-Two

Cam Derringer sat on his balcony, drinking a Belikin beer. He had his feet up on the railing, looking out over the moonlit sea and listening to the sounds of the surf. His thoughts drifted to Key West and his daughter Diane. When he arrived at the resort, he called her on his cell phone to let her know everything was fine. He did the same every morning and evening before bed, too. He was just getting ready to call when his phone lit up and rang. The screen said Nigel Logan.

"Well," he said, "is it good news or bad?"

"Don't be so negative, buddy. I have her."

"Where are you?"

"In the parking lot of your resort. We need a place to lie low for a while."

"Do they know she is missing?"

"Not until the morning."

"I'll be down in a sec. What are you in?"

"White Jeep. We're right out front."

Cam came out the front and looked around. "Dang," he said, "all the Jeeps are white." Then he saw one flash its headlights. As he approached, Nigel and Benita got out of the car. He extended his hand, and she took it. "Dr. Cabrera, I assume?"

She nodded.

"Dr. Cabrera," said Nigel, "this is my good friend Cam Derringer from Key West. The one I was telling you about."

"Thank you, Mr. Derringer. Mr. Logan told me how helpful you've been."

"And now, after finally getting to meet you, I can safely say, 'My pleasure.' Until now, I wasn't so sure. And please, call me Cam."

"Yes," said Nigel, "and again. We've been over it before. No more Mr. Logan. Call me either Nigel or Chief."

"Only if you will drop the doctor stuff and call me Benita."

"It's a deal."

"Come on," said Cam, "let's get inside. Are you hungry?"

Benita shook her head, and Nigel said, "Thirstier than anything else. Lead me to Jim Beam. It's been a long day."

They went to the room, and Nigel looked around. "Nice digs, my friend. Not a bad way to sit around and do nothing."

"I would love to complain, but..." Cam turned his attention to Benita. "Please make yourself at home. You must be tired."

She looked at the single king-size bed with concern.

"It is yours. I am sure the Chief and I will be up most of the night."

"Thank you," she said and got comfy on the mattress.

"Hey... Cam," said Nigel. "Come over here. I got something for you."

As he headed that way, Nigel pulled a bottle of Wild Turkey from a bag. "I don't have any chocolate-covered honey buns, so this will have to do." He looked over at Benita. She had her eyes closed. "Come on. We'll let her rest. Grab a couple glasses and some ice. We'll talk on the balcony."

Cam handed Nigel a drink and sat down. "So where are we?"

"I'm not exactly sure. Basilio has her kids. He's supposed to call me in the morning."

"And she doesn't have her passport?"

"No."

"And you never cleared in, so I can't get y'all past immigration and fly you out of here."

"You might not have to. He said he'd send for her. I'm not sure what that means."

"So, we wait."

"Yeah. We wait."

They sat looking out over the water. Cam was on his third drink, while Nigel paced himself and nursed his first one down to nothing.

"Want another?" asked Cam.

"Maybe just a splash."

Nigel watched and learned a Cam *splash* was really more like a double.

"Thanks."

"No," said Cam, "thank you. You're the one that brought the booze."

"That's not what I was talking about. Thanks for helping me and Benita."

"We are not out of this yet, so don't get all sentimental on me. I get nervous when you get mushy."

"Deal." They clinked glasses and heard the sliding glass door open. They turned to look. Benita stood in the doorway, holding a Belikin.

"I can't sleep. I'm too scared and excited."

Nigel got up and moved to another chair to make room. He patted his old chair. "I was just keeping it warm for you. Please join us."

And she did.

Chapter Thirty-Three

Morning came. Ernesto got off the bus in front of the marina. It was still dark. Sunrise below the horizon. He stood at the stop well after the bus had moved on. His eyes were closed as he tried to settle his nerves. Then he took a deep breath and exhaled it with a huff. He opened his eyes and said to himself, "Let's do this."

As he walked down the dock toward his boat, another fishing guide called out.

"Ernesto! Your charter is already here. He was walking the docks when I got to the boat."

"Oh... Thanks, Marco. Where is he?"

Marco turned and pointed the other way. "Over there. Big guy. I asked him if he was looking for a trip, but he said he had already booked with you."

"Yeah. I got the call late last night. I was planning on taking the day off, but he's willing to pay double. Wants a shot at a blue marlin. Maybe we'll have better luck than yesterday."

"You're funny, Ernesto. It wasn't a marlin, but your boxes were jammed full when you got back to the dock yesterday."

It's a different type of luck I need today, he thought. "Just wish me well. We'll need it. And I pray you'll book a trip today."

"Thanks!"

Ernesto turned to look at the man casually walking the docks and looking at boats. They'd never met, and he wondered if he really wanted to. Then he walked to his boat and was later joined by Paco, his trusted deckhand.

"I thought we were taking the day off?" asked Paco.

"Something came up, Paco. Another *special* trip."

"Ah. Those make me nervous."

"Me too, but we just have to do as we always do. It's just another fishing trip."

Paco nodded.

"Now get aboard and get the boat ready."

A while later, while checking the live well for bait, a powerful voice said, "Captain Ernesto?"

He looked up on the dock to find a man worthy of the voice. "Yes. And you are... Basilio."

"That is correct."

"So, you've been here for a while."

"That would also be correct."

"And your gear? I presume..."

"You would be three for three. Yes. Everything is stowed away and secured below."

"Very good. Let us set the poles out, rig the rest of the boat, and we'll get underway at first light."

When the white Impala came rolling down the street, Maria came bursting out of the apartment and ran toward the car. Bernard sped up to meet her. She was out of breath. Sam rolled down his window.

"Bernard! Sam! She is gone. I don't know where she is?"

"Dr. Cabrera?" asked Sam.

"Yes! Yes! Of course."

"When?"

"I don't know. Sometime last night. While I was sleeping, I guess."

"Get in. Maybe she's at the clinic."

Maria jumped in the back seat. "I hope so."

Bernard made quick time to get to the clinic. When they came in the front door, Maria called out. "Benita! Dr. Cabrera!"

The appearance of Yesenia, coming out from the back, answered her calls. The look on her face said all they needed to know. Then she said, "Come. We have a problem."

They followed her back to Dr. Cabrera's office. The desk had been cleared, and all the family photos were gone. "This is how I found it this morning. I've already called the Ministry of Health and the embassy."

Sam grabbed the phone and said, "I'll notify the office."

Bernard said, "It just doesn't make sense. Did you notice anything odd about her lately?"

"Yes," said Yesenia, "She has seemed nervous and distracted for the last couple of days. Wouldn't you agree, Maria?"

Maria shrugged her shoulders.

"Can you remember when it started?" asked Bernard.

Sam hung up the phone and joined them.

"Sure. Ever since the American came back. Seems like she has been on pins and needles from the moment he left."

"The American?" asked Sam.

She turned to leave. "Sure. Let me get his file."

She came back shaking the folder and dropped it on the counter. "His name is Nigel Logan. Had a nasty stingray barb deep in his foot. The doctor had to cut it out."

Bernard picked up the folder and quickly glanced at it, looking for anything that might help. When he turned the page, Sam pointed at the face on a copy of a U.S. military identification card. "Bernard. It's that Jim Horton guy that bought our breakfast." He looked at Yesenia. "What did you say his name was again?"

"Nigel Logan."

Bernard said, "And it's the same Jim Horton we saw hanging around Dr. Cabrera's apartment."

"Yes," said Sam. "And remember... he told us Dr. Cabrera removed a stingray barb."

"That's right," said Bernard. He turned to look at Maria. "Do you remember seeing him around?"

"No," she lied. "Just when he showed up for that follow-up visit."

"Damn!" said Bernard. "The embassy goons are going to be pissed. We need to find her first."

Yesenia said, "When I called the embassy, they said they would fly right down."

"He has to have a car," said Sam.

"Yeah," said Bernard. "Get on the phone and call the rentals. See if a car has been rented to a Logan or a Horton."

On the second call, Sam covered the mouthpiece on the phone. "Bernard. It's Koool Cars. They rented a white Jeep Patriot to one Jim Horton."

"Get the tag."

Sam waved a piece of paper in the air. "Got it."

"Good, get the word out and an all-points bulletin on that car. Plus, we need to check with the hotels. Maybe we'll get lucky."

Chapter Thirty-Four

Ernesto stood at the helm of the flying bridge and eased out into the bay like it was any other day in paradise. Paco swabbed the deck. Basilio sat in the big chair out in the open, taking in the sunshine. When a patrol boat roared by, Basilio gave a friendly wave. The driver gave an unenthusiastic wave salute. Ernesto picked up the pace but stayed behind the patrol at a reasonable distance. As they exited the channel, the patrol boat turned to starboard and traveled west along the coast at a high rate of speed. Ernesto eased to port and took on a southeastern bearing. He turned his head as he felt someone climbing up to join him.

"What can you tell me about those guys?" asked Basilio.

"What, the patrol? They have a routine. The two of them go up the Bay of Pigs to Playa Larga to have lunch and flirt with the bikinis. They'll be there all day."

"And the radar dome?"

"All for looks. Hasn't worked in years. No money."

Basilio pulled out a piece of paper, handed it to the skipper, and powered up his satellite phone. "Stand on that throttle and stay on this heading for another ten minutes, then set a course for these coordinates."

It was a little after ten in the morning when the embassy goons, Ramon and Cleto, touched down at the Placencia airstrip. They grabbed a taxi and went straight to the clinic to question Maria. She was strong in her defense of ignorance and told them what she knew. "They don't know for sure, but they suspect she is with a man named Nigel Logan. He goes by Jim Horton too. That's all I know. You should talk to the police. They are out looking for her now."

Ramon said, "Come on, Cleto. Let's go."

Cleto nodded, then turned back to Maria. "Don't you even think about doing something so stupid."

She visibly became angered and said, "I'm here, aren't I? I'm doing my duty for my country. Can't you see that? I'm not going anywhere. Now go find her!"

Cleto drew a hand back to slap Maria, but Ramon grabbed his wrist. "Cleto! What are you doing?"

"She can't talk to me like that!"

"And if you hurt her, you will have to answer to the brigade. Now, let's go."

Ramon and Cleto went to the station demanding an update from the chief.

"We know he stayed at Brisa by the Sea," said Chief Garbutt. "Checked in as Mr. Horton and checked out yesterday afternoon. Paid cash. Paid cash for the car as well."

"And what about the car?" asked Ramon.

"We have every jurisdiction between here and Belize City on the lookout."

"You're not doing enough!" shouted Cleto.

Chief Garbutt was much like Bernard and Sam. He cared very little for Ramon and Cleto. And if there is one thing he wasn't willing to put up with, it was having them tell him how to do his job. "If you raise your voice at me one more time, I can promise you I will call all my men off this case."

"You can't do that." snapped Ramon.

"I absolutely can. For one, as far as I know, she has committed no crime. If we find her, what am I supposed to hold her on? Not showing up to work?"

"What are you saying, chief?"

"Basically, she is not our responsibility. She is yours. Our Ministry of Health pays your country handsomely for her services. And if she won't work, Havana won't get paid."

"Are you threatening the agreement between our countries?"

"Not at all. I don't know that much about the arrangement. I really don't care. All I know is this… our community loves Dr. Cabrera. She is a fine doctor and very good to our people. I'm looking for her for that reason and that reason alone."

Ramon and Cleto said nothing but returned an aggravated stare.

"Now sit your asses down or get out there and help find her."

"They sat."

It was a little after two in the afternoon when Chief Garbutt's phone rang. It was Bernard. "What do you have?"

Ramon and Cleto sat up straighter.

The chief looked their way. "They found the car."

The goons sprung to their feet. "Where is it?" demanded Ramon.

Chief waved Ramon down so he could hear. "Okay. Good. Keep me informed." He ended the call.

"Well?" asked Cleto.

"Guys from the station in Dangriga found the car. It's in the lot at the Pelican Beach Resort. Local authorities will keep an eye on it until our guys get up there. They're on their way there now."

"Tell them to turn around and come get us," said Ramon.

"No," said the chief, "they are more than halfway there now."

"Damn you, Chief."

"Watch yourself, Ramon. I wasn't kidding earlier."

"Come on, Cleto. Let's go. We need a car."

Chapter Thirty-Five

Earlier that morning, when things were blowing up on the Placencia peninsula, Nigel, Cam, and Benita drank coffee and ate pastries that Cam had brought back from a small bakery a few blocks away. They sat on lounge chairs out by the water, so the satellite phone would have a clear view of the sky.

Things were quiet in Dangriga. For now, anyway. They looked out over the calm water. The sun was well up and warming the earth. The wind was calm and the water flat. Now and then, a small swell that had traveled hundreds of miles would make a five-inch curl and end its life on the sand.

"Did he say when he was going to call?" asked Cam.

"No. Just to keep the phone powered up and wait. I'm not crazy about sitting out here in the open. That's for sure."

Benita looked at her watch. "It's after nine. They really know I'm missing now. That's for sure. And I'm even more sure that Havana has been notified. God, I pray my children are safe."

Nigel reached over and took her hand. "I'll pray with you. I'm not very good at it, but I'm getting better."

All three of them closed their eyes and silently said their own version, requesting to be blessed with safety and success. Then the phone rang. Nigel got up to step away and answer it.

"Basilio. Where are we?"

"Where are you?"

"Hiding out in a seaside resort in Dangriga."

"How is the doctor?"

"She's scared, but ready to be united with her children. Is there a report I can share with her?"

"Tell the good doctor that the children are fine and excited to see her."

"I'll do that."

"Good. And you say you are by the seaside. That is fantastic. Do they have a dock or pier?"

"As a matter of fact, they do. A big one. It's quite long."

"Even better. Do you feel good about this place? Are you safe?"

"I guess so."

"Again, good! When we hang up, text me your GPS location."

"Will do."

"In the meantime, stay low and stay put. I am sending a boat, but it won't be there for a while. Should arrive around three or three-thirty."

"Okay, how will I know which boat? They come and go all the time."

Basilio laughed. "Trust me, my friend. Monitor the time window, and when you see it, you'll know. You will make a joyful sound and say, 'Ha! Only Basilio.'"

Nigel said nothing.

"Okay, my boy. Got to run. See you soon." And the call ended.

Nigel walked back with a smile. "Benita. Basilio reports the children are doing fine."

"What else?" asked Cam.

"He's sending a boat. It will get here around three or three thirty this afternoon. Till then, we keep a low profile."

After the call, time seemed to stand still. Very still. Watched water never boils. That adage certainly proved its point. All three sat on the balcony and they did their best to take their minds off of the situation, but it was impossible. Small talk didn't help.

"Well, Cam," said Nigel. "I guess you'll be flying home without me. If we didn't need the room, I'd say that you should probably head on out. I know Diane is probably chomping at the bit to get you home."

"Even if I could, I wouldn't leave. I'm not going anywhere until I know you and Ms. Benita are safely out of here."

"Thanks, man. I appreciate it."

Then a new distraction came along. Nigel's phone bonged with a text message. He looked at the screen. *Damn.* It was from Red.

Are you getting this? Thought I would try your phone. Haven't heard from your Spot thingy since you entered the gulf.

The last thing that Red knew, Nigel was on his way home. Nigel usually sends updates and positions so folks can gauge his progress and keep up with the trip. Obviously, that wasn't happening.

Nigel studied the screen. He read the text repeatedly, trying to decide how he wanted to reply. Being big on honesty, he decided the best reply, at the moment, was no reply at all.

"Who is it?" asked Cam.

"Ah, just an old friend from St. Joe. Checking up on me."

"Speaking of checking up," he said, "have either of you checked your watches and appetites? It's almost one-thirty, and I for one am getting hungry. Forget *getting*, I am hungry."

Benita said, "I have to admit, I'm feeling a little empty."

"That's all I needed to hear. I'm going out for sandwiches. Are you in, Nigel?"

"Yeah. Anything is fine."

"Same here," said Benita.

Cam left and ordered sandwiches at a little deli he had found around the corner. He was gone maybe thirty minutes. As he walked back, he halted in his tracks before crossing the street to the resort. Three police cars surrounded Nigel's Jeep. *Oh shit. Not Good*, he thought. Then he took a deep breath and crossed over to where the police were standing around the car. It was time to play nosey tourist.

One cop saw him coming and took several quick steps to meet him halfway. "That is far enough," he said.

"Sure. What's going on?"

"Nothing, really. We're looking for the person driving this car. He may have a female companion with him. You don't happen to know anything about it, do you?"

Cam stuck his bottom lip out and shook his head. "Nope. Have you checked with the front desk?"

"Yeah. The driver and the car don't appear to be registered here."

"Oh, so you know who you are looking for?"

The cop unfolded an enlarged copy of a picture of an ID card. "We're looking for this guy. It's not a very good picture, but have you seen anyone around that resembles him?"

Again, Cam. Shook his head.

"Here is a picture of the woman. Have you seen her around?"

Cam was still shaking his head. "But… I'll keep an eye out. Is the guy dangerous?"

"We're not sure, so I wouldn't approach him if you come across."

Cam nodded and walked away. *You're not sure, huh? I'd want to be… if I were you.*

Cam made sure he wasn't followed and went back to his room. He shut the door and said, "We have a problem."

"What?" asked Benita.

"The noose is getting tighter. Local cops have the Jeep surrounded."

Suddenly, the hunger pangs were gone.

"You're kidding me," said Nigel.

Cam returned a, *Would I kid about such a thing*, look. "I spoke with them. They have a bad, enlarged picture of you from your military ID. I don't think they would recognize you if you walked right by, but the six foot three, two hundred thirty-pound description might tip them off. Benita, they have a perfect picture of you."

"My ID? How the hell?"

"The clinic," said Benita. "We would have made a copy of the card for ID and insurance purposes."

"But we paid in cash."

"Doesn't matter."

"That's right. Y'all filed a claim. I remember now."

"I don't know about that. That's Yesenia's responsibility."

Nigel walked over to the sliding glass door. "I wonder how they connected me to you?"

"What do we need to do?" asked Cam.

"Damn," said Nigel as he peered out from behind the balcony curtain. "They're searching the grounds."

Benita asked, "Did you see anybody else with the police?"

"Like whom?"

"Men in suits, not in uniform."

"No. Why?"

"Men from the embassy. If they're not here now, they will be before long."

"What kind of men?" Nigel asked while secretly watching the search efforts.

"Terrible men. They won't let me go anywhere if they get their hands on me."

Nigel turned to look at her. A familiar tingle of adrenaline filled his senses. He walked toward her. She looked worried and more scared than ever. Tears filled her eyes. He smiled as he took his thumb and pushed an escaped teardrop to the side. "Now stop that. Everything is going to be alright. Trust me."

There was a quiver in her voice when she said, "But you don't understand."

Nigel smiled even larger, and from across the room, Cam said, "No. *They* don't understand."

Nigel turned to his friend with a look.

"What?" said Cam. "They don't… right?"

Then came a knock at the door.

"Mr. Derringer. It is the manager. Please open the door?"

"Umm… Sure, hold on! Give me a second!"

Cam looked at Nigel and Benita, then pointed to the bathroom. As they slipped inside and closed the door. Cam gave a look out the peephole. Yes, it was the manager and two other men in plain dress. The knocking started again, and Cam opened the door. "How can I help you?"

"May we come in, please? We would like to have a word."

"What is this pertaining to?"

One man held up a picture, obviously from surveillance footage. It was of himself, Nigel, and Benita as they were returning to the resort after Nigel's phone call.

"I don't understand."

Nigel felt like an idiot. The bag with the Ruger sat out on the balcony. He kept his ear close to the door to listen.

"Where are they?" asked the other one.

"I do not know," lied Cam. "I only met them yesterday. They are staying here, somewhere."

"No, they are not," said the manager.

The two other men held up identification for Cam to study, and one of them said, "We need to search the premises. Please step aside."

Cam did and raised his voice. "You can look, but there's nothing to find."

With weapons drawn. One looked around the room and balcony. Nothing. The other checked the closet. Nothing. Then he opened the bathroom door.

Nigel found himself with a revolver pointed at him. He was on alert and ready to attack. Benita was behind him, with her face buried behind his back.

Nigel's built-up adrenaline and fury were milliseconds away from going on offense. Then his target smiled.

"Mr. Horton. We meet again." He leaned to the side to speak to Benita. "Dr. Cabrera, has he harmed you in any way?"

Benita lifted her head, recognizing the voice. "Bernard? Is that you?" She looked around Nigel. Both Bernard and Sam stood before her.

Bernard repeated the question.

"No, dear God, no. He is helping me." They lowered and holstered their weapons. "We've missed you, Dr. Cabrera," said Sam.

"I'm not going back. I'm not."

"You might not have a choice," said Bernard.

"Oh! Trust me," said Nigel. "She has choices, and they all belong to her."

Bernard and Sam turned and went into the room. "Please, come out so we can talk."

They left the bathroom. Nigel looked at Cam, who shrugged his shoulders.

"Why?" asked Sam.

"Yes," said Bernard. "Help us understand. We thought you liked it in Placencia."

"I do. The people are so kind and friendly."

"Those people think highly of you, too."

"I know, but..."

She looked at Nigel and could tell his nerves were on end.

"They are friends, Chief. It's okay. You can calm down now."

"Easier said than done, Doc." Whenever his heightened senses take over, they are tough and slow to abate. He knew the sensation all too well, so he looked at Cam and said, "Where's the Wild Turkey?"

Benita explained her circumstances. That she didn't come to Placencia of her own free will. Both Bernard and Sam were shocked at what they heard. They knew that she and Maria were on loan from Cuba, but they didn't know the rest of it. Then, when she came to explain the death of her husband, Alejandro, they both stood. "You gotta be kidding me," said Sam.

Nigel said, "She's not. It is state-sponsored human trafficking. The Cuban regime profits dearly on their services, and severely punish those who resist. They have no choice. They're trapped. But she's not. Not anymore."

Sam got up and walked away. "I can't believe this. And you say you're to be united with your children?"

Bernard looked at his favorite doctor.

She nodded. "Yes, after over four years."

"Dammit!" said Sam. "So, Mr. Horton, what's the plan?"

"We leave by boat. It's supposed to be here between three and three-thirty."

"Simple enough," said Bernard, "except for two things."

"Cleto and Ramon," said Sam.

"Who?" asked Nigel.

"The guys from the embassy," said Benita.

Bernard looked at his watch. "They got to be getting close. They were, what, probably forty-five minutes behind us?"

"At normal driving speed, yeah," said Sam. He thought for a second, then said, "Well, yeah!"

"What is it?" asked Nigel.

Sam smiled, grabbed his phone, dialed his boss, and went out onto the balcony. He saw some uniforms still walking around. The phone answered. "Hold on, Chief." Then he called down to the ground. "Hey! You guys!"

The uniforms looked up.

"We got her. All good. Thanks for all your help. We got it from here."

One of them called up. "Are you sure, Sam? We can stick around."

"It's all good. Just a misunderstanding. We're all clear."

Sam watched the back courtyard clear and walked back into the room. "Chief, are you still there?"

"I am. So, you got her?"

"Yeah, but we don't have time to explain. Please, as soon as we hang up, call Ramon and tell him we got her and to call me to arrange a place to meet, so we can hand her over."

"You want to turn her over to them?"

"Not exactly," said Sam. "We'll have to explain later. Just call them for us." He listened some more, then finished the call. "Thanks, Chief. We'll be in touch."

"Brilliant," said Bernard.

"Exactly," said Sam, "those goons have no reason to believe we're not cooperating." He looked at his watch. "It's two forty-five. I hope that boat is early and not late."

Sam's phone rang. "Here we go." He pushed the flashing green button. "This is Sam." He listened, looking around the room at everyone. "Yes. Yes. Yes. We have her. You can slow down. How far out are you?"

"Fifteen minutes?" Sam rolled his eyes. *Come on boat!* "No. The locals caught up with them. They were down at the marina on Gra Gra Lagoon, looking to hire a boat." He listened some more. "We were just getting ready to leave here. Sure..." He winked at Bernard. "... we'll wait. Then we'll escort you to the Dangriga airstrip to take her back to Belize City. Don't worry. Everything has been handled. See ya in a while." He hung up the phone.

"That will take them in the opposite direction," said Sam.

"For a while anyway," said Bernard. "But when they get there and find nothing. Boy are they going to be pissed."

Sam walked back to the balcony and pulled back the curtain. "Come on, dammit. Get here."

Nigel walked up to look out the sliding glass door, too. "Thanks. I can't tell you..."

"Then don't. It's unnecessary. Turns out we are on the same team."

"We don't want to lose her, but we care about her more," said Bernard. "The whole town does. Once they learn the truth, they'll understand."

Cam looked at his watch. "It's five till. You two better get on down there. When that boat shows up. You gotta hightail it out of here."

"What about you?" asked Sam. "Are you going with them?"

"Who me? Nah. And by the way, I'm Cam Derringer. I seemed to have been left out of the introductions."

"So, you're not getting on the boat?"

"Nope." He looked over at the resort manager, standing quietly in a corner the whole time. "I was hoping to extend my stay, if that is alright with you."

"Yes, sir. How long?"

"A week perhaps."

"But Cam," said Nigel, "What about Diane and getting home?"

"My friend. As soon as I stand on that balcony and watch your boat disappear over that horizon. I'll make arrangements for Diane to meet me here. We both need a vacation."

Nigel smiled. "Well played, buddy. Just remember, one thing, once I'm gone... you're off the financial tit."

"Agreed. Now you and Benita get your asses down on that dock."

While Cam, the resort manager, and Nigel chatted. Benita said her goodbyes to Bernard and Sam. Not a dry eye between the three of them. Then Nigel said, "Come on doctor, we got to go."

She sniffled and wiped her eyes. "As you say, Mr. Logan."

Chapter Thirty-Six

The marina was bustling with activity when Ramon and Cleto arrived. They drove through the parking lot looking for any sign of Bernard or Sam. Nothing.

"Where are they?" asked Ramon.

Cleto looked at his watch. It was seven after three. "Call them. Find out where they are."

Ramon opened his phone and dialed. It rang and rang with no answer. As he listened to the ringing, he said, "I don't like this."

Cleto pointed. "Over there. Come on."

Across the parking lot sat a Dangriga squad car. A uniform was leaning up against the fender. Ramon and Cleto pulled out their identifications and showed them.

Ramon read the name tag on the uniform. "Officer Santos, we are looking for the two officers from Placencia. They have the man and his female companion your department helped to apprehend. Where are they? We're here to take custody of the woman."

"Do what? What are you talking about?"

"The man and the woman. The ones y'all found looking to hire a boat."

"Mister, I've been here... Oh, wait. The guys from Placencia and the white Jeep. That wasn't here. That was in town at the Pelican Beach Resort. They found them there. I listened to it all on the radio. It's all good. Some misunderstanding or something... Hey! Where are y'all going?"

They ran back to their car as quickly as their feet would allow. Ramon yelled, "I can't believe this! Pull it up on your phone! Get directions."

They were speeding back toward town. "Seven kilometers and seventeen minutes away."

"I'll do it in ten!"

Nigel's eyes were focused on the water and horizon. No boat. He looked at this watch. 1521. *Dammit.* Then, from somewhere, a distant roar filled the air. Nigel looked over the water. Nothing.

From his balcony, Cam pointed up in the sky and yelled, "Nigel! Look!"

But the roar was too loud. The noise sucked Cam's words in.

He didn't see it at first because he was still focused on the water, but as the roar got louder and louder, it became obvious. It was behind him… and ABOVE HIM. He turned around and looked up. "You have got to be kidding me."

A big Grumman Albatross flew above, just above the treetops. It headed seaward until it banked hard and circled around for an approach toward the long dock. Nigel watched as it kissed the water, sending a mild spray. Then it settled down, plowing and splitting the gentle waves. When it became apparent the flying boat was planning to dock, several staff members ran to help tie it up.

Nigel laughed.

"What is it, Chief?"

"Only Basilio."

Nigel turned around and saw Cam. He was giving a big thumbs up. He turned to Benita. "Come on."

They walked out on the long dock and kept their distance as the plane was secured. With the engines winding down, the side door opened and a guy, well-tanned with shoulder-length hair jumped out to help secure it. He wore a colorful tie-dye Columbia fishing shirt with the top two buttons missing, a medallion of sorts hung from around his neck. He had on khaki shorts, and flip-flops. Moments later, a young lady appeared and stepped out on the dock. Then a boy.

Benita covered her mouth. "Oh, my God. Lucia! Antonio! Thank you, Jesus." When the three of them saw each other, they broke out in a run and met halfway. Benita fell to her knees, crying as her children smothered her with hugs and kisses.

Nigel watched the reunion and pushed away a few tears of his own. He tilted his head and looked toward the heavens. *Thank you*.

He turned his attention back to the threesome and smiled. They really needed to get going, but he didn't want to interrupt them. And, at that moment, Benita didn't care; she finally had what she had longed for. To see her children. She was so caught up in the joyful moment that she never noticed the other passenger step off the plane and walk toward her, but she looked up when she heard her name.

"Papa? Oh, my God! Papa!"

She stood, ran to him, and she fell into his embrace.

"I am so sorry, Benita."

"Hush, Papa. Hush. We'll talk later."

Earlier that morning, after the embassy in Belize City called Havana, they dispatched MININT to the home of Fredrico to check on and collect the children for safekeeping. Colonel Garcia banged on the door. No answer. He looked at his men. "Break it down."

They did, and the colonel entered first. The main room was empty. Rope and wadded up balls of duct tape littered the floor. "Search the premises," he ordered. It did not take long for the small house to declare itself empty and person-less.

One soldier in the kitchen called out, "Sir. Over here. A note for you."

Garcia took the folded piece of paper, unfolded it, and studied the writing.

Colonel Garcia,

You have made a grave mistake in your judgment. Not even you can keep me from fulfilling my wishes. As you read this, know that my family is free and safe. But you, on the other hand, will never be safe. I will continue to lurk in the shadows behind you. Trust me on that, as I swear on the name of my grave.

Alejandro Cabrera

The evening before, as Basilio was about to leave, Fredrico was secured, gagged, and looking at the floor in defeat.

"You know Fredrico. It doesn't have to be this way. There is nothing here to stay for. The country you think you love betrayed all its people long ago. You are just too old and stubborn to see it. This is your last chance. I hate breaking up families. It's my least favorite thing to do. Come with us, so you can be with your grandchildren and love your daughter. Because, once I'm gone, you will never see them again. So, what will it be?"

Slowly, the realization hit him. *Never* was not just a long time. It was *forever*. He raised his head. "And it is a better life?"

Basilio smiled. "Like no other."

While the reunion was in full swing, Nigel slung his bag over his shoulder and walked past them to give them space and talk to the guy who emerged from the plane. "I gather you're our pilot?"

"That's right, and we have to get a move on."

Nigel reached out his hand. "I'm Nigel Logan."

"I gathered that. Basilio was pretty clear in his description. The name is Buck. Buck Reilly. Listen. We got to go."

"The sooner the better."

"I'll fire up the engines again. Please, go break up that little party and start loading them on board."

As Nigel spoke with the pilot, Sam and Bernard were standing guard in the parking lot. Ramon and Cleto came in hot with a gravel-sliding halt. They got out and ran to Sam and Bernard.

"You sons of bitches!" yelled Ramon. "Where is she?"

"You're too late. She's gone. We took her to the airport and put her on a plane," said Sam.

"Impossible!" yelled Cleto. "She has no identification or passport."

"This is Belize, Ramon. We have friends."

The timing couldn't have been better. The Dangriga Airport is only a short distance away and the single airstrip points out to sea. As if planned for the moment, a turboprop from Maya Air took off and flew overhead, heading out over the sea.

"There she goes."

As the plane banked north, another roaring commotion from behind the resort shifted everyone's focus.

"What is that?" demanded Ramon as he started toward the resort. Cleto was close behind. Then a second roaring commotion joined in with the first, and the embassy goons drew their weapons and broke out in a full sprint. Bernard and Sam were hot on their heels. When they came around the corner of the building, they saw the big flying boat. People were boarding.

"There she is!" yelled Cleto.

Ramon yelled, "Stop! Stop! All of you, stop!"

Watching from the balcony, Cam said, "Shit!" Then he left the room to go out toward the dock.

Their words were faint in the cacophony of the two Wright R-1820 engines, but it was enough for Nigel to turn around and look.

"Dammit." He turned to Benita. "Hurry. Get in and tell the pilot to get out of here."

"No. I can't leave..."

But Nigel had already taken off in a run. As he ran, he unslung his bag and opened it. He reached in, withdrew his Ruger Mark IV, and dropped the bag.

Cleto was much faster than Ramon. He had a significant lead as he sprinted down the dock. As Cleto closed in, he fired two shots in the air. "Stop! Get out of my way!"

Nigel, with his weapon hanging by his side, slowed and stepped to the side. He gave the plane a quick look. Benita was still standing there. "Get on the plane!"

She didn't.

The resort staff no longer helped and jumped into the sea to swim to shore, so the pilot came out to untie the plane. He yelled at his passenger. "Get on board!"

"Dammit," said Nigel. Then he turned his attention to the first guy running.

To Cleto, it appeared Nigel stepped aside to allow the man to pass. It was really to set the poor fool up for the worst closelining of his life.

As Cleto drew near, Nigel clenched all his muscles tight, stepped in, and quickly reached out and swung his arm, catching Cleto's Adam's apple perfectly where the humerus and radius come together to form the inside of the elbow.

The acrobatics were impressive. Cleto flipped backward. The back of his head struck the dock first. Shocked and stunned, his weapon came out of his hand, and Nigel kicked it in the water.

One down, he thought. Nigel turned to look at the plane. "Benita! Get on board!"

She shook her head.

Shit!

As he turned his attention to the next guy, he heard her say, "Not leaving without you!"

Dammit! Nigel took a firm stance, lifted the Ruger, and painted the guy's forehead with the red dot from his optic laser sight.

Ramon slowed down to a walk and did the same.

"Stop right there," said Nigel.

He did, five yards or so from Nigel. Bernard and Sam took up positions behind Ramon with their weapons drawn.

"Drop the weapon, Ramon. Now!" yelled Bernard.

Ramon ignored the demand. "Step aside. It isn't a request. This is official business. Dr. Cabrera is Cuban and works for the government. She cannot leave."

"You Cubans have a strange definition of employment, and besides, she gave her resignation. She quit." He turned his head to the side. "Benita. Please get on the plane and go."

"No," she said.

"You are a smart woman," said Ramon. "Now come with us."

She said nothing.

Nigel sized up his adversary. He was a big fella. Not as tall as himself, but he had a firm build with plenty of muscles. He looked capable and his tight, square jaw gave an air of competence. A worthy adversary.

"Benita," said Nigel. "If you don't get on that plane, I will be forced to kill this man. And neither you nor I, and I might guess..." Nigel stopped to address the man standing before him. "What did you say your name was again?"

Ramon said nothing.

"... our friend here want anything to do with dying today. So, please, get on the plane, I will be fine. The gentleman and I are just going to have a little talk."

Nigel never took his eyes off his target, lowered the Ruger, and said, "What do you say, pal? Let's talk." Nigel turned his weapon away from everybody and released the clip, catching it in his other hand, then he pulled the slide bolt back and ejected the chambered round. As he slowly squatted down to place his weapon on the dock, he said, "What do you say, buddy? You wouldn't shoot an unarmed man? Talk to me."

"There is nothing to talk about."

Nigel stood and took a couple of steps forward. "Oh, sure there is. You see, you're in a bit of a pickle."

"Stop! And how do you figure?"

Nigel stopped and spread his arms out. "You could shoot me now, and it would suck and hurt, but I'd most likely live. I've had practice. You, on the other hand, probably not."

"You make big talk."

"No, just sensible talk. If you were to be so brave as to shoot me, Sam and Bernie..."

From behind the Cuban came, "It's Bernard! Bernard! Not Bernie."

"My apologies, Bernard. Anyway, if you shoot me, Sam and Bernard will have no other choice but to fill you with lead. And it would be all for nothing because whether or not you kill me, Ms. Benita is getting on that plane. Sam and Bernard will make sure of it. Won't you boys?"

"Absolutely," said Sam.

"Without question," said Ramon.

"Gosh. I hate not knowing your name. Bernard? Can you help me out?"

"It's Ramon. The other one is Cleto."

Distant sirens could now be heard over the plane engine. The resort manager called the police at the first sound of gunfire.

Nigel turned for a quick look at Cleto. He was on his belly now, still lingering. "So you see, Ramon. I don't want to get shot. You don't want to die. And it doesn't matter, because you lose either way. Sucks doesn't it. Makes you want to take a swing at me, huh?"

Nigel smiled as he watched Ramon's face build with anger.

"Chief!" said Sam. "You don't have time for this. We have him covered. Just turn around and get on the plane."

"Sam's right," said Bernard. "We got this."

"I'd rather he drop the weapon first, boys. And if he does, he knows you guys won't shoot an unarmed man. Then I'm pretty sure he'll want to dance and have that little chat." Nigel gave Ramon a wink. Then he puckered up and blew him a kiss. "Come on, sweetie. I'll let you pick out the music."

Ramon dropped the handgun and charged Nigel, yelling.

Nigel got Ramon's jaw with a solid right hook, but Ramon still tackled Nigel and drove him down on the deck. As they hit the boards, Nigel used their momentum to lift a leg and flip Ramon off. Nigel got to his feet. So did Ramon, and they squared off. Nigel quickly learned that his assessment of his opponent being worthy was accurate. A quick and well-placed left hook sent Nigel staggering. Then a blow to the stomach sent him to his knees. Ramon took another swing at the side of Nigel's head, but a quick dodge found Ramon scoreless. As his fist found only air, Ramon felt his groin being sent to his ears. He clutched over and was helpless. Nigel struck Ramon two more times where his hand tried to protect his jewels.

Nigel got to his feet. His target struggled, but got up and remained bent over. It was the perfect opportunity to end everything, so he lifted his knee into Ramon's face, sending him backwards. Nigel stood over him.

"Get up, dammit."

Cam was watching from the beach. Then several Dangriga police officers arrived and ran down the dock toward the action. Cam followed.

When Sam heard the commotion behind him, he looked and waved the other officers down.

To Nigel's surprise, Ramon slowly got to his feet to square off again. They circled, going around and around. Then Nigel channeled his old mentor, the grade school janitor, Mr. Wilson. *What would you do? What would Mr. Wilson do?*

The answer came as a second-nature instinct.

Ramon came at Nigel with a big, swinging left hook.

Nigel ducked for the miss and immediately went inside with three fast punishing blows to the left kidney. As he backed out, Nigel tagged him with a left jab. It backed him up, so Nigel hit him with another and another. Ramon swung and hit Nigel several times, but the blows had little to no effect. Then two quickly applied right hooks sent Ramon to his knees. The last uppercut drove Ramon on his back. He was done.

Nigel stood over him for a spell, panting. Then turned to look at Sam, Bernard, and everybody else on the dock.

They watched Nigel walk around, out of breath. He found his bag, then retrieved the Ruger and clip. He put them in the bag and stood looking at Sam and Bernard.

Nobody said anything.

When Nigel turned around to get on the plane. He found Cleto staggering on the dock. When their eyes met, Cleto surprised Nigel when he raised a .38 caliber revolver and pulled the trigger.

Nigel fell to his knees, then to his side.

As the pilot hit the deck and with Benita curled up in a ball, Sam and Bernard both fired three shots into Cleto's center mass. He swayed back and forth, trying to walk, but found the edge of the dock. He went over the side. Sam ran over to check. Cleto was floating face down.

Benita ran to Nigel and rolled him on his back. Others quickly joined them.

He looked up at her and whispered, "Can we leave now?"

"You need medical attention."

"I thought you were my doctor."

She unbuttoned his shirt and pulled it back. "He got your left shoulder."

"That's where it seems to hurt the most."

"Can you roll over so I can see the back?"

He did.

Then she gently rolled him back. "No exit wound. The bullet's still in there. Can you move your shoulder at all?"

Nigel winced and gritted his teeth as he gave it a rotation and a small lift. "Yeah, it hurts like hell, but I'll take a gunshot wound all day long over a stingray barb."

Benita smiled and helped Nigel to sit up.

Nigel looked around and found Cam's face smiling down at him. "Hey, buddy. Thanks for all your help earlier."

"Don't mention it. I thought you were doing okay by yourself until that last part."

"Sure."

Bernard looked at Benita. "Dr. Cabrera, is he okay to travel?"

"I think he'll be fine. I'll be with him."

"Good, because y'all need to get going."

An aggravated Buck Reilly said, "It's about damn time. Let's go."

Benita turned toward the pilot. "You have a good first aid kit, correct?"

"Absolutely. Now let's get a move on."

The lead Dangriga officer said, "Leaving? Nobody's going anywhere! Somebody needs to tell me what just went on here."

Sam said, "We'll explain everything. It's complicated. But for now, you guys need to trust us. The doctor and..."

Sam looked at Nigel.

"Mr. Horton."

"Yes. The doctor and Mr. Horton need to get a move on."

Buck helped Benita aboard. Before Nigel ducked his head to go in, he said, "Thanks for waiting."

"You can thank Basilio. He said, 'Buck! I can't make any promises, but if you can get them out of there, I'll see if I can't do something about that little problem you have with the FBI.'"

"What's that mean?"

"Long story. Just get on board and get comfy. Takeoff is going to be quite bumpy. Your shoulder ain't gonna like it at all."

"I'm sure I've had worse. Let's go."

Chapter Thirty-Seven

As *Big Mama* transitioned from boat to plane, the southern waters off Cienfuegos, Cuba, were abuzz with patrol boat activity. Additional boats had been dispatched to search for every vessel on the water. As the bikini-chasing officers made their way back, they spotted the vessel *Mare Stella* and made a beeline for her. As one officer drove, the other grabbed the binoculars. He dialed in his focus and reported. "She is going astern!"

The one driving looked at his partner.

Onboard *Mare Stella*, Paco was coaching Basilio. "Easy now. Don't overpower him."

Basilio dragged the pole to a vertical position, then quickly lowered it, cranking on the big Penn reel to take up some slack. Sometimes Basilio would make gains. Sometimes the big fish would take it back from the drag setting. It was a take and give and give and take situation.

"The fight has just begun. Let him wear himself out. Be patient," said Paco.

Basilio nodded. He looked at the deckhand. "Big fish."

Paco smiled. "Yes."

From the flying bridge, Ernesto said, "Mierda! We have company."

Paco looked in the direction his skipper was pointing. The boat was up on a plane and moving their way fast. The deckhand waved his arms in the air, then tried to wave the boat off. Paco pointed to the big man in the chair fighting the big fish, then out toward the water. The boat kept coming and finally slowed and followed to keep pace as *Mare Stella* moved astern, trying to follow the fish and reduce the pressure on the fishing line.

The driver of the patrol boat spoke through the radio and onboard PA system. "We have to search your boat!"

That's when the Spanish yelling started. Ernesto yelled as he tried to pay attention to what was going on behind the boat. "We are a little busy here. It will have to wait."

"We don't have to wait."

"Then go find somebody else to board. Can't you see my charter has a great fish?"

"We are coming aboard."

"You have got to be kidding me!"

Basilio was oblivious to what was going on as the patrol boat maneuvered in. He stayed focused on the fish until he felt the two boats gently collide. Surprised, he turned his head to look and saw the uniform jump aboard.

Paco scolded Basilio. "Pay attention! Pay attention!"

He did, turning back to study the progress he was making on the fish.

The patrol officer looked up at *Mare Stella's* skipper as the patrol boat eased away and stayed close.

Ernesto yelled at the officer. "Do what you have to do, but if I lose this fish. I swear!"

The uniform disappeared down below. He was only down there for a few minutes before coming back up on deck. He looked over at his partner and shook his head. Then he looked in the boxes on deck. One was the livewell, full of bait. The other contained a nice dolphinfish. He turned his attention to the man in the chair and wanted to ask his name.

The fish was making its way around to starboard, toward the officer.

As Basilio rotated his chair to stay in line with the fish, Paco yelled at the officer. "Get out of the way!"

He did.

Moments later, the big blue marlin broke the surface of the water to show itself. Its tail danced across the water as its head tried to shake the bait loose.

Basilio let out a boisterous, "WHOOO! HOOOO!"

The officer walked around to the other side and waved his partner over. In short order, the pilot of the patrol boat retrieved his partner.

"Nothing?" asked the pilot.

"Let's go. As we suspected, there's nothing there."

Ernesto paid no attention as the two gave a little salute. Then the driver stood on the throttle and whisked away.

Once they were in the air, Benita took off Nigel's shirt and gasped. Buck heard her and turned to look. "How is he?"

"He'll be fine. It's just..."

"Just what?"

"Nothing really. He's fine."

Nigel looked up at Benita's pretty face. His voice was tight with tension from the pain. "What has you troubled?"

As she held pressure to the wound with one hand, she took the fingers of her free hand and gently touched Nigel's other scars. "Dear God in heaven. How many times have you been shot and stabbed?"

"I don't know. A few. I don't keep score." Then he smiled. "It seems to have become a bad habit. Can you get it out? The bullet, that is."

"While we are in the air? I think not. I don't have everything I need, plus..."

"Please. I'd rather you do it now."

"Forget it."

"But you don't understand... If I go home with a bullet in my shoulder... seeking medical attention. That would be no good. There is no way to explain it, and all it will do is open up a huge can of worms."

Benita looked confused. "A can of worms?"

"It's an expression. Trust me, we need to get this thing out before we land."

As she slowly shook her head, Nigel called up front. "Buck, is there any booze on board?"

"Rum."

"I'd like to buy it from you. Ms. Benita and I are going to need it."

With the plane on autopilot, Buck left his seat and brought a full bottle of Papa's Pilar Flagship Dark. He unscrewed the cap and handed the bottle over.

Nigel looked at Buck. "Nice sipping rum, but there will be little sipping today." He took a long pull off the bottle. The burn felt good. He took another pull and swallowed, then offered it to Benita. "Please, you have to do this."

"I don't want to. Not here."

"Please."

Benita took the bottle and took a sip. Then another. Then she handed it back to Nigel, who turned it up once more for another long draw. She looked at Buck. "Will you help?"

"What do you need?"

"Get that first aid kit and help keep him still. That will be a tremendous help."

Benita was impressed with the supplies that were on the plane. It wasn't perfect, but it was better than most. Once the rum had taken its desired effect, she took the bottle and hit hard to settle her nerves. Then she poured some on the wound and a pair of hemostats. She handed the bottle back to Nigel and asked, "Are you ready?"

He took another deep swig, swallowed, and nodded his head.

She went straight to it and worked the hemostats into the entry wound. Given Buck's size, he had no problem holding Nigel down, who had closed his eyes, clenched his teeth, and tried to stay still and shake as little as possible. The search had just begun.

Chapter Thirty-Eight

An hour later, Benita was in the back of the plane enjoying her family. It was impossible to catch up on everything they'd missed over the past four years, but it wouldn't be for a lack of trying.

Buck was back behind the controls as the plane flew itself. Nigel sat opposite him, patched up, holding tight to an empty bottle of rum, and sleeping.

Later, as Nigel stirred, Buck noticed his eyes flutter. "How are you feeling?" he asked.

Nigel squinted hard and looked at the bottle. "Like I haven't felt in a long while." He put the bottle down and shifted in the co-pilot seat to get comfortable. A piercing pain shot through his shoulder. He felt the bandage with his free hand. "Did she get it out?"

Buck looked at him. "You don't remember?"

"I don't remember crap."

"You're gonna have the *rum-dumbs* later. Here, hold your hand out."

He did, and Buck dropped the slug in his palm. "Damndest thing I ever saw."

"For me? How sweet of you." Nigel brought it up for closer inspection. "The son of a bitch shot me. Can you believe that?"

"I saw it with my own two eyes." From under his seat, he produced another bottle of rum. "My emergency stash. Want a nip?"

Nigel shook his head. "Would you happen to have Diet Coke on board?"

"'Fraid not. Sit back and get some rest. We're going to be in the air for a while."

Nigel nodded and closed his eyes.

Nigel remained asleep for a long time. Never even batted an eye as the plane touched down in Cancun for refueling. About an hour outside of Cancun, he felt his shirt being opened. He opened his eyes saying, "Candice? Is that you?" As his eyes came into focus, he saw Benita, playing Dr. Cabrera and checking on her patient.

"Who is Candice?" asked Benita.

He gave her question serious thought and said, "Nobody. Not anymore anyway."

Benita gave a huff of disbelief and said, "Your wound is looking good."

Nigel smiled, and she smiled back.

"Thank you for taking such care of me," he said.

Benita turned her head to look back at her father and children. "No," she said, "thank you. You have given me back my world."

She put a hand on Buck's shoulder. "That goes for you too, Mr. Buck."

"My pleasure, ma'am."

She snuck in and gave him a peck on the cheek. Then she turned to Nigel, cupped her hands around his cheeks, and pulled him in for a long kiss on the forehead.

Nigel blushed and said, "Go. Be with your family. I'm fine."

She did, and he held his breath as he watched her move aft with the grace of an angel.

"Is it true?" asked Buck. "The things Basilio told me about her."

"I'm not sure what you know, but yes. I'm quite sure he wouldn't lie about it."

"The Cuban government executed her husband?"

"Yes. Bastards."

"She seems to be a remarkable woman."

"That she is."

They were quiet, and Nigel was still. The pain in his shoulder was increasing. Then Nigel said, "Change of subject. Where is Basilio? Why isn't he on the plane?"

"He was supposed to join us. But when we got the kids and the old man aboard, he gave me your coordinates and told me to take off without him. That he had unfinished business."

"What unfinished business?"

"Said he was going fishing. That there was a big marlin in his future."

"You're kidding me. We're getting our asses shot at, and he's gone fishing. Only Basilio."

Buck laughed, and Nigel tried, but his shoulder would have nothing to do with it.

"So, how are we doing this?" asked Nigel.

"Doing what?"

He used his thumb to point over his shoulder. "Getting them into the States."

"Ah, there is a boat waiting. We'll land and rendezvous. Then it is up to them to do whatever and however they get it done. Then you and I will return to Key West."

"Sounds like a plan." Nigel looked out the window. The pain in his shoulder was real, and the Motrin that was onboard could only do so much. Plus, he was thirsty. "Do you have anything onboard to drink?"

"Oh, crap. I'm sorry. I forgot." Buck reached down into a cooler and produced a Diet Coke. "Here. I picked a few up while we were refueling."

"Oh! Bless you, my child." He popped the tab on the can and took a drink. "Thank you."

"You're welcome."

Nigel pointed. "That. What's that around your neck?"

Buck pulled out his necklace. "A Spanish real."

"A what?"

"A Spanish Escudo… pure gold."

"Oh! Nice. Replica?"

Buck laughed. "No, it's the real deal."

"That had to set you back a sweet penny."

"You could say that. In the end, it was worth every cent. I found it."

"You what?"

"Found it. I'm a treasure hunter. It's what I do."

"Really?"

"Ever heard of the company e-Antiquity?"

"Can't say I have."

"Well, in its heyday, people knew me as..."

"What?"

"Nothing. That was a long time ago. Today my partner and I run Last Resort Salvage and Charter."

"I gather the salvage part is for the treasure," asked Nigel.

"Yeah. The business has its ups and downs."

"And when it's down... you charter."

"We got to keep the bills paid."

"You fly folks around for Basilio?"

Buck looked at Nigel and said, "Every now and then."

"Hey," said Nigel, lifting his one good hand in the air. "Full disclosure here. I know what Basilio does, and I'm not judging."

"Trust me. It's safer helping Basilio than hunting treasure. Plus, I get to eat for free in his restaurants."

"Why do you do it?"

"Like I said, 'to keep the bills paid.'"

"No. Treasure hunting."

Buck looked at Nigel. A sincere seriousness stretched across his face, and with no emotion at all, he said, "It's an addiction. Stronger than anything you'll ever know."

Nigel believed him and felt it best not to pursue the discussion further. Buck appreciated that.

Nigel finished his DC and tried to subject himself to more rest and, hopefully, sleep. Sleep would take his mind off the pain. He closed his eyes, and though sleep never came, he rested. After a while, Buck made an announcement. "Grab a seat and buckle up. We'll be landing soon."

The visibility wasn't great. A ceiling of clouds made seeing anything below impossible, but as the plane came out of the coverage, the water came into view. Buck banked the plane and pointed. "There she is. Right on time."

"Where are we?" asked Nigel.

"About 90 miles southwest of Sanibel Island."

"Oh, that far north?"

Buck said nothing.

Nigel looked out the window as the big, deep hull closed in on the Gulf of Mexico. Then, just before the hull kissed the water, Buck said, "Hold on, folks." It was a painful landing for Nigel, but still a thrill. As the plane became a boat, Nigel said, "That was pretty cool."

Buck smiled. "Water landings are my favorite. Come on."

Buck unbuckled himself and Nigel. Then he went aft, opened the hatch, and waved at the Grady-White Freedom 375 as it slowly made its approach. Luckily, the sea state wasn't too rough, so they transferred everybody without too much trouble. Benita was the last to debark *Big Mamma*. She said her goodbyes to Nigel.

"Get to a doctor as soon as you can. You hear me?"

"I will. Don't worry."

"Will I ever see you again?" she asked.

"I don't know. If I had to guess, I would say, 'yes.' After all, you're my doctor now, right?"

She smiled, and he kissed her on the cheek. "Get out of here. Adventure awaits."

She gave him a quick and gentle hug that made him wince. Then jumped on the boat.

As the Grady-White backed away, Buck waved. Benita and the kids waved back. Her father didn't, as he was still unsure about what lay ahead.

"She's still looking at you," said Buck.

"Yeah, and I'm still looking at her."

"Is there something going on here?"

Nigel stopped waving, slapped Buck on the shoulder with his good arm, and said, "Nah. Don't be silly. It's just..."

"Just what?"

"Nothing. Come on. I miss my sailboat."

As Buck was shutting the hatch, he said, "What kind of sailboat?"

Chapter Thirty-Nine

When they landed in Key West, Buck taxied toward his hangar while Nigel pulled out his phone. The screen was dark, so he tried to power it up. It offered a quick effort as the screen glowed, then it faded back to certain death. "Shit."

"What?"

"Phone's dead."

"What about the sat phone?"

Nigel powered up the Iridium. "Sure, it works, but what good is that if you don't know the number? Who remembers numbers anymore?"

"I barely remember my own. Who do you need to call?"

"My Uber driver."

"You have an Uber driver?"

"Yeah, Teddy. Well... sort of. He drives for Uber, but I call him directly. He picks me up and I pay him cash."

Buck pulled out in front of the terminal and shut down both engines as another guy ran out toward the plane.

"Where do you need to go?"

"To see a doctor. My shoulder is killing me."

"Don't you think showing up in your condition is going to be like throwing a spanner in the works?"

"It could, but it hurts like hell. Plus, I have a plan."

"I'll take you wherever you want to go."

"Thanks."

The back hatch opened.

"Buck," said the man, "everything go alright?"

"We're home aren't we? And we got paid."

"Good! We need the money."

"Nigel," said Buck, "this is my partner, Ray Floyd. Ray, this is Nigel Logan."

"Nice to meet you," said Ray. "Oh, Buck... by the way, Agent Booth keeps calling. He's mad as hell that your phone's been off."

"Lovely. Did he say what he wanted?"

"He said, 'Your ass,' if you don't call him back."

"Perfect. Thanks for the good news, Ray. Nigel, grab your things, and we'll get moving."

"You know the address?" asked Buck as they rolled down Eaton Street. "That would help, you know."

"I'll know it when I... There! Up ahead on the left."

Buck stopped out front.

Nigel reached out with his good hand, and they shook. "Thanks for all your help. Maybe we can meet up for a drink. I owe you a good bottle of rum."

"Not necessary. And please, don't take this the wrong way, but I hope we never meet again."

Nigel nodded. "Yeah, probably for the best."

Nigel got out and Buck Reilly wasted no time exiting, stage left.

"Do you have an appointment?" asked the receptionist. Giving him a good once over, she suggested, "Perhaps you need the ER."

"No appointment and I've already been seen at an ER. Sort of. I'd like to see the PA, Dr. Juan Cruz."

"We'll have to work you in. What is the need? I'm guessing the shoulder."

"Yes." Nigel opened a few buttons and pulled back the corner of his bloody shirt. "Shoulder injury."

"Have a seat."

"Thank you. May I ask another favor?" He lifted his Samsung. "My phone is dead."

"Sure. Let me have it."

Two and a half hours later, he was called back and put in a room. Five minutes later, PA Cruz knocked, then entered with a folder in his hand. He stopped to look at his notes. "It's Chief, right?"

"You remembered. Very good."

"What can I do for you?"

Nigel finished unbuttoning his shirt and fully exposed the blood-soaked bandage. "Perhaps a dressing change and something for the pain."

PA Cruz helped Nigel remove the shirt. "When did this happen?"

"Yesterday."

"Well, let's take a look." The PA stood next to Nigel and began unwinding the bandage. "So, what exactly happened?"

Nigel never blinked and kept his eyes trained on his face. "GSW."

The PA stopped what he was doing and stepped back. "A gunshot wound. You must be kidding."

Nigel slowly shook his head.

"Do the authorities know about this?"

Nigel kept shaking his head.

"Well, I must call them at once."

Nigel's head never stopped shaking, slowly and methodically.

"Why not? And where did this happen?"

"Because it's complicated and Belize."

PA Cruz said nothing.

"Doc, do you remember the last time I was here? I spoke of the doctor who helped me down there. When you discovered she was with that Cuban medical brigade operation, you became visibly upset. Do you remember?"

"The brigade is awful."

"I know. I've come to understand that. So, all I can tell you is... that doctor, Benita Cabrera, she is now safe and removed from any regime control or danger."

"You mean that you..."

"I mean nothing. Just know that she is safe, happy, and reunited with her family. It was mighty compassionate that you showed concern."

The PA said nothing.

"And this thing hurts like hell."

Fifteen minutes later, Nigel and his caregiver walked out to the reception counter.

"Sally," said the PA, "we are done here."

"Very good," she said. "Chief, here is your phone. Is it the same insurance?"

"Thank you, yes, and wow, I like this place." He turned to the doc and offered his hand. "Thank you, sawbones."

"You're welcome, Chief. And please, be more careful with that nail gun."

"Pretty stupid, huh?"

"Beautifully stupid."

Out on the front porch of the clinic, the same rooster and iguana were waiting on him out on the railing. Or, at least, they looked the same. He sat on the steps and powered up his phone. After connecting with the network, a musical barrage of bongs and dings flooded the air space, notifying him of missed text messages and calls. He looking at them. Most of the texts and missed calls were from Red. He opened and read the last text.

I know you are not coming home. And I don't like what I see. You are scaring me.

Nigel looked at the time stamp. "Crap," he said aloud. "He knows."

Red is a lot more than Nigel's best friend. While his outward appearance might not always express it, he is intelligent, with special talents. A couple of years back, he started searching for his inner self to find enlightenment. He now alleges the ability to see images and have visions. Nigel has always dismissed such nonsense, but, if pressed for honesty, he cannot deny the uncanny things he has witnessed from Red's talents.

Nigel rubbed his head and sent a simple reply.

Hey, buddy. It's all good. I'm fine.

It took all of three seconds. *Bong!*

I guess you're going to say... It's complicated.

Nigel didn't reply.

One of the missed calls was from Candice. It came earlier that morning. He felt his heart race a bit. Then, he saw she had left a voicemail and his heart skipped a beat. He hit play.

Hey Nigel. Red said you were coming home the other day. Folks were excited. Then, yesterday, he told us not to expect you. I thought I was looking forward to seeing you, too. Now, I'm not sure. Anyway, be safe out there.

Nigel deleted the voicemail and said, "Thanks for the help, Red. Nice job."

Then he went into his contact list and hit the green dial button. It rang three times.

"Chief! How are you?"

"In need of a ride, Teddy."

"But I thought..."

"That's your problem... thinking. Come get me."

Chapter Forty

Nigel sat on stool 17 at Navigator's, sipping a Diet Coke. What a long, exhausting day it had been. He looked at the bartender. "Hey, Steve. I appreciate you picking me up at the gate."

"No problem."

"How have things been around here?"

"Quiet and slow."

"Good!" said Nigel. "I'm ready for some quiet and slow."

"So, are you going to tell me what happened to your shoulder or not? You know I won't stop asking."

"Really, Steve. It's not a big deal."

Steve returned a deadpan stare. He's quite familiar with Nigel's past. Maybe not so much of the more recent history, but the beginnings for sure and how Nigel can be a magnet for trouble. He kept staring.

"Okay, dammit. If you must know. It's embarrassing. I was helping a friend, you see, and there was this nail gun, and..."

Steve threw his hands in the air. "Just stop. I know the feeling of hot smoke getting blown up my ass, so just stop."

"Steve... that sounds kind of personal, like a little too much information. I'm not so sure I would share..."

"Just shut up. Forget it. I don't want to know."

Bong!

Nigel checked his phone, stared at the screen, opened the text, and smiled.

Hello friend.

Nigel got up. Tossed three bucks on the bar and said, "Steve… saved by the bong."

When he got outside, he hit the dial button. The call was answered in one ring. "Hey, baby. That was quick."

"I can be when I need to."

She said, "I like you when you're slow."

"I can do that too."

"I know and I miss you. Where are you now?"

"I miss you too," said Nigel. "What if I told you I was actually in Key West?"

"You are kidding me."

"Nope."

"I want to see you."

Nigel looked at his watch. "I want to see you too, but I can't be sure when. But I promise, it will be as soon as possible."

"Beggars can't be choosers."

"I will not lie. I like it when you beg. Sweet dreams."

"Oooo, you just gave me a quiver. Good night."

The next day, he showed up later than he or she wanted, but certain things had to be handled first. Rest being one of them. It was just after seven in the evening when the Uber driver stopped in front of the house. Nigel handed his driver a twenty and said, "Thanks," before getting out.

After the car left, he stood out in front for a while.

Then the front door opened. She stood at the door wearing tight blue capri pants and a white silk blouse. Several top buttons were already undone. In her bare feet, she strolled down to the sidewalk where he stood. She wrapped her arms around his neck. She felt him wince and backed away, but he grabbed her by the waist.

"It's only a flesh wound." Then he pulled her into a long, wet, passionate kiss. When they came up for air, she said, "I missed you, Florida Man."

"I've missed you too, Sherry Stone. I was pleasantly surprised to get your text yesterday."

"I'm crushed. Have you already forgotten our little annual arrangement?"

"Sort of. I've been a little preoccupied." Nigel looked at the house, around the yard, and driveway, looking for evidence or a sign. "So… what about Felix?"

"He's no longer around. Probably a good thing."

"I'm sorry," said Nigel. "It seemed y'all were getting along."

"I don't want to talk about Felix." She gently touched where she could see the bundle of bandages under his shirt. "High adventures, I presume."

"You could say that."

"Another damsel in distress?"

"You could say that, too."

"Well, let's go in. You can tell me all about it."

"Not now. I want to go in and talk about something else."

"Well… my, my. Look who's begging now."

Chapter Forty-One

The relationship between Nigel and Sherry Stone goes way back to the beginning of Nigel's troubles in Norfolk, Virginia. She was the television news reporter following the murder case, and she provided him with insulation and protection when none of the other news reporters would. They barked like hounds. She gave him space and earned his respect and admiration. A deep and affectionate relationship grew with only one obstacle that stood in the way: Nigel's girlfriend, Candice. At the time, he was still deeply in love with her. And as years passed by, Stone was always there as a friend. Later, after Nigel rescued her from the grips of evil monsters, they ended up rescuing each other. Once Candice pushed Nigel away, he and Stone became special long-distance lovers with a unique problem. She was promoted to the morning news desk as an anchor and couldn't leave Virginia. He had deep roots in Florida and couldn't leave the sunshine state, though those roots seem to get shallower.

After the surprise phone call with Stone, Nigel called Cam.

"Hey, buddy, want to log some more flight hours?"

"Ah, my initial reaction is no, but what are you talking about?"

"I need to get to Virginia as quickly as possible. Strictly personal, not business. If you know what I mean."

"No can do, my friend. Don't you remember? I stayed in Belize. Diane flies in tomorrow for a few days."

"Crap! Are you saying…?"

"Yep… you better call Priceline or Travelocity."

"Cam, I could be in the air all day."

"Sorry, pal. I know there are two direct flights daily that go into Atlanta. I'd shoot for one of them."

"So much for having a personal pilot."

"Have a pleasant trip. OH! By the way, there is this outstanding local rum called Big Titties. Have you ever heard of it?"

Nigel rolled his eyes. "Enjoy your stay, buddy. You're wasting my time."

As Nigel arrived at the residence of Sherry Stone, a weary and still frustrated Colonel Garcia ended his day, as he always does, with cocktails and dinner at Villa Maria in downtown Cienfuegos. As he entered, there was a man and woman sitting at a table, and two men at the bar. The owner and bartender, Alex, greeted the colonel.

"Buenas noches, Señor Colonel. Good to see you again. The usual?"

"Gracias, Alex. Si."

The colonel took his usual seat toward the back, facing the door. Alex delivered the cocktail and a menu. "Does the colonel know what he wants to eat tonight, or would you like the menu?"

"Leave the menu." He looked around and commented, "Slow night?"

"Si, colonel. It has been a very busy week, so… no complaints. Just let me know when you would like to order."

After a spell of studying the menu, the colonel caught Alex's eye and gave a little motion to come.

"Yes, señor?"

"I'll have the Ropa Vieja with the normal sides."

"Ah, so you decided on the usual after all. Very good."

As Alex made casual chitchat with the colonel, a man entered the restaurant and took a seat at the bar. Alex turned his head. "I will be with you in a minute, señor."

The colonel leaned over to look around Alex and see the stranger.

The colonel sat up straighter and asked, "Who is that?"

Alex turned his head to examine the customer and shrugged his shoulders. "Don't know. Never seen him before. Is there anything else I can get for the colonel?"

"Not at the moment."

"Very well."

Alex went to the bar, placed the order in the kitchen window, rang the bell, stuck his head in the window, and yelled inside an empty kitchen. His cook staff had already been sent home for the evening with pay. "Order in!"

Alex turned to his new customer and never said a word. He placed a glass in front of him, then reached under the counter, produced a bottle of seven-year-old Havana Club, and popped the cork. The customer poured a healthy amount into the glass, then turned around to sip and take in the room. When the colonel made eye contact, the customer raised his glass and said, "To Castro."

The colonel raised his glass but said nothing.

After a few minutes, the stranger got off his stool, took his bottle and glass, walked to the colonel's table, and sat down uninvited.

"What is the meaning of this? Who are you?" demanded the colonel.

"It isn't who I am that is important. It's who you are."

"Leave my table at once!"

The stranger smiled, then took a long sip of his rum.

"I'll tell you one last time. Leave me."

The stranger's smile turned sour, his eyes squinted, and through his teeth said, "Bastarda."

The colonel slid his chair back, stood, and reached for his sidearm. As he did, the two men at the bar and the man at the table stood and drew their own guns and pointed them at the colonel. The woman calmly got up and left the restaurant.

The colonel looked at Alex, expecting support, but found a stare that told him he had none. Then the door opened and another man that Garcia didn't know entered. Alex joined the new customer, closed all the blinds, and hung a sign on the door. *Closed for a Private Event.*

The new stranger joined the party at the table. The bottle of rum was handed off, and the new stranger said, "Gracias, Montego."

The colonel spoke up. "I am Colonel Garcia of MININT. I demand to know what is going on."

The new stranger took a long draw off the bottle and said, "You surprised me, colonel. I would have never expected the tough and terrorizing Colonel Garcia to be drinking a Mojito, a little girl's drink."

The colonel said nothing.

Another pull was taken from the bottle, then he said, "I imagine introductions are in order. This gentleman is Montego Cabrera. He's the brother of Dr. Alejandro Cabrera, the man you executed in the cemetery in Palmira. And I am... Nigel Logan from the United States."

The colonel scowled. "You do not look like someone that would be named Nigel."

"You are correct. I lied. If I were going to allow you to live, I would try to convince you of that name, but since I am not..."

"Who are you?"

The stranger put down the bottle, walked around, and relieved the colonel of his sidearm. Then he walked back around and handed the weapon to Montego.

"WHO ARE YOU!"

"You know who I am, or at least you should know my name. I'm Basilio. Basilio Valdez."

The colonel looked down and up to search his memory. The name sounded familiar, but from where?

"Come on, colonel. Think! Remember!"

Then Colonel Garcia's head snapped back to look at Basilio. "The smuggler! Basilio Valdez the smuggler!"

"I prefer Basilio the exporter... but call it what you will. Now you understand why I can't let you live."

An anger grew in the colonel, and he growled, "What do you want?"

Basilio smiled. "I want to welcome you to the resistance!"

Early the next morning, Captain Ernesto and Paco arrived at *Mare Stella* sooner than usual. They stopped at the boat together and looked around the marina before boarding. Nothing seemed out of the ordinary.

Paco said, "Let me guess. Another special charter?"

"Si. Get the boat ready. He will be here soon."

"Very well. Is there any reason for me to go below?"

Ernesto looked around and found what he was looking for. An empty bottle of Havana Club sat on the deck by the salon door. "No. I'm sure it is secured for sea. Get the poles. I'll check the boxes."

"Aye, aye."

Ernesto cautiously walked aft and stood before the big fish box where they store the daily catch. He held his breath and opened it to look inside. It seemed they had already caught the day's limit. A wide-eyed and severely bruised face of Colonel Garcia lay looking up with cold, dead eyes. A trickle of blood oozed from a single gunshot wound from between the eyes. He closed the box and became startled when he heard the words, "Captain Ernesto?" He spun around, "Si."

"I am Montego Cabrera. I am your charter for the day."

"Yes, that's what I understand. I'm glad you are here. Please climb aboard. Paco and I are eager to get underway."

"As I am."

"Paco! Forget the poles for now. Our charter is here. Cast off the lines."

It was five-thirty in the morning and Nigel was still asleep. Sherry Stone was next to him on her side, stroking his chest. *Sleep baby, sleep.* She slid out of bed to go downstairs and make coffee.

Stone winced and looked to the ceiling as the loud Keurig machine coughed and gurgled the last bit of water in the cup. She added heavy cream, as that was the way she now took her coffee, thanks to Nigel. Carefully, she went up the stairs, trying not to make too much noise, and went back to the room. Nigel was still out. She put the coffee down and pulled the covers up around his neck. He smiled briefly as she let go of the covers. She drank her coffee from an easy chair across the room and watched him peacefully sleep, feeling grateful that he was back in her life, for whatever time they had left. With a whisper she said, "I still love you, Nigel Logan."

Ten minutes later, he stirred, and she got up to sit on the side of the bed. His eyes did a brief flutter, and he looked at the ceiling, trying to get his bearings.

"How do you feel?"

He turned his head. All she had on was the unbuttoned silk blouse. He reached out, and she took his hand. "I was feeling like shit until I saw you sitting there. Now I feel much better. What time is it?"

Stone turned away to look at the clock. "A quarter to seven. You slept straight through. Unusual for you."

He stretched as much as his shoulder would let him, and said, "Give me a little credit. I'm trying to turn over a new leaf."

"Coffee?"

He looked over and saw her cup. "Any left?"

"A little less than half a cup."

"That should be enough to get rid of this sticky morning mouth."

She brought it to him. It was lukewarm, but still good. When he finished, he placed the cup on the nightstand and pulled the covers back to display his state of preparedness. "Join me."

She did, gently crawling into bed and easing a leg over him to straddle his hips. When she was settled, he reached up with his good hand and removed the silk blouse. He gently brushed his fingertips over her breasts, and she responded with a quick twitch.

"You are beautiful," he said.

Stone leaned forward, being careful about his injury, and placed her elbows on either side of his head. She kissed him.

When she finished and pulled away, they gazed into each other's eyes for a while.

"Stone?"

"What, Chief?"

"I still love you, too."

She pulled back her head a bit. "Did you hear me earlier?"

"I thought maybe I was dreaming."

"No. You weren't."

They kissed again, then Stone asked, "Why do our lives have to be so complicated?"

"I don't know. Believe me, I'm trying to uncomplicate mine."

"I can't see that happening anytime soon, but sleeping in until almost eight is a good start."

"Baby steps, Sherry. I need to take baby steps."

"Say it again..."

"Baby ste..."

She placed her fingers over his mouth. "Nigel Logan... Don't ruin this."

He smiled. "I love you, Sherry Stone. Is that what you want to hear?"

She smiled and nodded her head. "Now show me."

Stone positioned herself and helped Nigel find his way, and as she settled upon him, she gasped.

As Nigel and Sherry resumed their panting, nearly thirteen hundred miles away, Montego rolled the body of Colonel Garcia over the stern of *Mare Stella.* Basilio followed with a forty-three-pound Danforth anchor that was tethered to his ankles.

Ernesto and Paco stood on the flying bridge, keeping a lookout with binoculars as Basilio and Montego chummed the waters.

"Good riddance, you bastard," said Basilio.

"It doesn't bring my brother back."

"I know. But at least justice has been served. Hopefully, that will bring you some closure."

"I hope so."

"Me too." Basilio called up to Ernesto. "Anything?"

"Nothing yet."

Basilio nodded, and he and Montego stood quietly for a long spell.

"There!" yelled Paco. "They are coming."

Ernesto fired up the engines, getting ready.

Moments later, an enormous shadow covered the deck. Basilio looked up with a squinting smile as *Big Mama* flew overhead and started its bank to begin its approach for a landing.

"Montego. I'd ask you to come, but I don't enjoy breaking up families."

"I understand. As tempting as it is, I feel I will be more effective here with the resistance."

Basilio nodded, and they turned to see the flying boat part the waves and settle down into the sea.

"Basilio... do you ever think we'll get our country back?"

"Keep the faith, my brother. It's in my prayers every day."

The big Grumman slowly taxied its way toward the boat. Ernesto piloted his vessel to rendezvous. Basilio saw the pilot's window was open, so he yelled, "King Buck! What took you so long?"

A middle finger was produced out the window as a reply.

"Ha, my friend! Good to see you too."

Chapter Forty-Two

Two weeks later, Nigel and Stone were having dinner at one of their favorite restaurants, The Orapax, in the Ghent section of Norfolk. The Greek fare was exceptional. Nigel dropped his fork on what was left of his salmon. "Oh, my God," he said, "just as I remembered. Consistently great."

"That's how they've survived for over fifty years," said Stone.

They were quiet and looking into each other's eyes, both smiling, when Stone broke the silence.

"I have to ask, you know... How long will you be staying?"

"Already trying to get rid of me, huh?"

She replied with a swift kick to his shin.

"Damn!" He reached under the table to rub his lower leg. "What did you do that for?"

With a sour puss look, she said, "It was my answer to a stupid reply to a serious question." She leaned forward and reached out with a hand.

He took it with the one not massaging his shin. Then he brought the other hand up and leaned forward too. "That kind of hurt, you know."

"Sorry, and stop being a wuss. I'll make it up to you later." Then she took his other hand. "I love you being here, but I know..."

"I love being here, too. And to tell the truth, I don't know when I'll leave. I guess I'll hit the road when I tire of your bitching."

"Do I bitch?"

"Only when I leave the toilet seat up. Other than that, no. Which means I may be here for a while."

She smiled. "I would like that. But I know better."

"I know, and I wouldn't be honest if I didn't admit that Florida pulls at me. The problem is, which Florida? Key West was temporary, but I've found it has been good for me."

"And St. Joe?" asked Stone.

"St. Joe is home, but I'm not sure it will be the same. But between the two, St. Joe is the magnet that pulls the hardest."

"And Candice?"

"Did you have to bring her up?"

"Well?"

"She is done with me. I'm sure of that. And..." He gave some thought to what he would say next, and said, almost convincingly, "I am sure I'm not interested in that drama anymore."

"Hmm! And what about in Key West?"

"What about it?"

"Is there a girlfriend down there?"

"Sherry. We've always maintained that our separate lives are just that, separate."

"And they are. I'm just a curious cat."

"There is a companion. A good friend. Let's leave it at that."

"Fair enough."

He said nothing.

"Aren't you at all curious about me?"

A call on Nigel's cell interrupted the line of questioning. He looked at the screen: Basilio. Before answering, he looked at Stone and said, "I think I'd rather not know." He pressed the green button. "Basilio. How are you? I guess it is safe to say you are back."

Stone listened to the one-sided conversation.

"I'm in Virginia visiting a special friend."

Nigel looked down at the table, then up at Stone. "We were just talking about that. I'm not sure."

He rubbed his head. "Tomorrow? No. I wasn't planning on..."

Stone's eyebrows lifted.

"Okay. But what does that have to do with me?" Nigel pushed his chair back and stood. "Why can't she talk to me over the phone?"

He sat back down. "Okay. Okay. Not tomorrow, though. The day after. I'll let you know my flight times."

Nigel listened some more. "Okay. Bye."

"Well, it sounds like you're leaving sooner than either of us expected. What is going on?"

"That was Basilio. The guy I told you about. It seems Dr. Cabrera has decided about her future and wants to talk about it with me."

"What does she want to do?"

"I don't know. They wouldn't say."

"So?"

"Well, you heard me. I will go back the day after tomorrow. Then I will fly back here, if that is okay with you."

"You are welcome here anytime, but I'm guessing you won't be back."

They held hands across the table and looked into each other's eyes, thinking the same thing. *She was probably right.*

Nigel jumped in the back of the Uber.

Teddy turned around. "Welcome home, Chief. Where to?"

"Lower Matecumbe Key. The Real Habana restaurant. And can we press it? I'm running a little late."

"I'll press it as hard as island time will allow."

"That's all I can ask."

Little was said between Nigel and his driver. Nigel spent most of the time looking out the window. Deep in thought.

When they arrived, Teddy asked, "Need me to stick around?"

He got out, paid, and tipped his favorite driver. "No. I don't think so. Thanks for the lift."

He walked up the steps and met the receptionist at her station just outside the front door.

"Reservations?" she asked.

"No. I'm here to see Basilio."

"Ah, you must be the Chief."

"Yes. And thank you for getting it right the first time."

She smiled. "Follow me."

They walked through the dining room. He looked at his watch. 1820. He was twenty minutes late. She led him out to the back veranda. All the tables were empty but one. Nigel saw Benita smiling at him when Basilio got up to meet him. Everyone else had their backs to him. Basilio and Nigel hugged.

"I'm glad you are back, safe and sound," said Nigel. "I gather you will tell me what happened down there."

"Yes, but not tonight, my friend. We have other business to discuss. Come. I think you know everybody." Everybody stood and turned around.

Nigel chuckled when Desiderio took a few steps to meet him. "I gather my satellite phone is safe."

"I'm happy to see you too, Desi. And yes, I have it here in my bag." Nigel fetched it.

Desi held a hand up. "No. Keep it. And keep it charged. You never know."

"I don't think I like the sound of that."

Nigel turned his attention toward the two other men that had stood. Nigel looked at them but spoke to Basilio. "What is going on? What are they doing here?"

The two men approached with their hands out. "Chief," said the first one. "Good to see you again."

The other one said, "We never had much of an opportunity to thank you or say goodbye."

"Bernard. Sam. You were the last two people I expected to see here today." Again, Nigel asked Basilio. "What is going on?"

"Perhaps it would be best if Dr. Cabrera explained," said Basilio.

Everyone took their seats except the doctor. Nigel walked around the table to where she stood. She was more beautiful than ever. No stress. No drama. She looked calm, free of tension, confident, and content as she took one of his hands and placed the other gently on his wound. "How is the shoulder?"

"Still sore, but getting much better."

She took his other hand, and they held each other's gaze for quite some time before she pulled him into a sweet kiss on both cheeks. "Hello, Chief."

"Hello, Benita. How are you?"

"I am fine and much better, thanks to you. It is so good to see you again."

"You look fantastic, and I really like this smile you have on. It's one I haven't seen yet. Keep it."

"I will try, but it may be up to you."

Nigel looked at Basilio, then back to Benita. "I don't understand. What is this all about?"

"I'm going back."

"To Cuba? I don't think so."

She smiled. "No, never again. Belize. The children and I are going to Placencia, where I belong, and I'm needed. It is what I want to do."

"But what about MININT, the brigade, and the embassy?"

"It's been taken care of, sort of," said Basilio. "Personally, I think she is crazy for not wanting to stay in America."

"Basilio," she interrupted, "I can't practice medicine in the U.S. You know that."

"I get it. I get it," he said. "Nigel, when she convinced me of her stubbornness, I got in touch with the Ministry of Health in Belize City. I explained the situation. They are thrilled for her to return. They will provide her with a special visa so she can stay and work. It will be more cost-effective to pay her than the brigade, and she will, for once in her life, make a decent wage."

Nigel gave it all a thought. "Passports? What about travel papers?"

Desi raised a hand. "That's been taken care of, too. Replacement passports have been issued."

"So Belize is going to kick the brigade to the curb?"

"Yes. And they are happy to do it," said Basilio.

"But wait! What about the nurse, Maria?"

Benita reached out and grabbed his arm. "She has been taken care of as well. As of yesterday, the country has severed its ties with Cuba and the brigade."

"Havana and the embassy are going to be pissed."

"They already are," said Desi. "They want Maria back, but she is in hiding until all this blows over."

Nigel stood and paced the floor. "I don't like it. I can't ever see it blowing over."

"It will take some time, but it will," said Basilio. "I've sent word to Havana that unless they want more MININT agents to die, they will stand down in Belize."

Nigel turned to Benita. "Are you sure this is what you want?"

"Yes."

"And what about your father?"

Basilio laughed. "Oh, he is adjusting to American life just fine. Turns out he loves it in Miami, and he can visit Benita and the children anytime."

"Okay," said Nigel. "So, what does any of this have to do with me?"

Benita said, "Please, sit with me."

He did and turned his chair toward her, and she turned her chair to look into Nigel's eyes. Now she held his arm with two hands. "I want you to come back with me. Stay with me and Maria until things calm down. Bernard and Sam are here to escort me back, and they will protect me when they can, as will the entire police department. But... I would feel much safer if you were with me at night."

"Ah, I don't know. I mean..."

"Please. I don't want to worry or be scared." Her eyes cut right through him. And the things that raced through his mind made him feel uncomfortable and distrust his willpower and intentions. "I just don't think it is a good idea."

She leaned in and kissed him on the lips. It was an innocent kiss, nothing sensuous or sexually explicit but a kiss, nonetheless. "Please," she said again. "Just for a little while."

"How long do you think?"

Basilio chimed in. "Probably six weeks or so."

Sam spoke up. "We would appreciate you being there, too."

"Yeah," said Bernard. "Just for a while."

Nigel looked again at Benita. She hadn't yet taken her eyes off him. He slowly nodded his head. "Okay. I'll do it. For you. I'll do it."

She whispered, "Thank you, very much."

Nigel kept nodding, thinking about only one thing. *Behave boy. You're going to need to behave*. Then he said, "I can do it."

"Do what?" asked Basilio with a crooked smile on his face.

"Oh, nothing. I got this." *I think*.

The End

Thank You

If you enjoyed *Trapped*, there are a few things you could do to make this author incredibly happy.

First, provide a short, honest review at Amazon. Those reviews mean so much more than you could imagine. It doesn't have to be long. We appreciate *star only* reviews too.

Second, if you like Nigel Logan and the gang, please consider signing up for my monthly newsletter. There, you will gain some insight into Nigel Logan and the knucklehead that created him. Oh... That would be me. PLUS! You can grab a **FREE** copy of *The Cuban,* a Nigel Logan novella I wrote just for you. And... If you join us, I will make you this one promise: *I will not fill your inbox with junk and SPAM.* Sign up at www.KirkJockell.com

And the third thing is, contact me. I love to hear from readers. Let me know what you thought of the book. It would make my day more than you can imagine.

Email: Kirk@KirkJockell.com
Facebook: www.facebook.com/KirkJockellAuthor
Website: www.KirkJockell.com
Book Bub: www.BookBub.com/Kirk S Jockell

Acknowledgements

My most sincere appreciation goes out to so many people. None more so than my wonderful wife, Joy. She is my bride, my partner, my rock, and number one supporter. To do things without her would be impossible. Her love and encouragement are nothing short of amazing.

Special thanks go out to two of my Tropical Author brethren: Mac Fortner and John H. Cunningham. They graciously agreed to have their characters, Cam Derringer and Buck Reilly, play significant roles in the story line. If you haven't started their series, I highly recommend it. Find Mac at: Tropical Adventure Series And John at: Buck Reilly Adventure Series

During my journey as a writer, my friends (old and new) mean so much to me. They provide the greatest support imaginable. There are too many to mention, but you know who you are. Thanks so much! You help to keep the engine running.

Getting emails from readers is one of the best parts of this job. Thanks to all of you that have done so. They are more valuable than the royalties. Words cannot express the appreciation I have for each of you. Thanks to you all!

Then, there are the folks that keep me from looking too stupid, which isn't easy. That I can promise. The editing and proofing team: Jan Lee, Tim "Coach" Slauter, Sandra Russel P'Poole, Frank Rush, and Lynn Story. Thanks, guys. We did it again.

About the Author

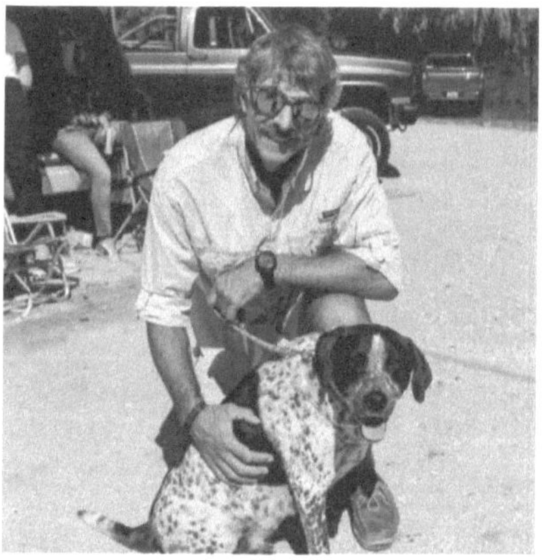

Kirk Jockell is an American writer and the creator of The Nigel Logan Action Series. Port St. Joe, Florida is home, but he sleeps many nights in Flowery Branch, Georgia, where his wife continues to work that regular job she loves. He patiently awaits the day she can join him in retirement and trade the daily grind for a simpler life back down on The Forgotten Coast. Kirk is a sailor and enjoys his 1991 Catalina 34, *JoyRide*. He loves to race sailboats, fish, throw his cast net for mullet, listen to music (Pop Country doesn't count), play his guitar, and drive his Bronco on the beach. Kirk lives with his lovely wife Joy, a rescued bluetick Apalachicola coonhound named Nate (#98Nate), and a tuxedo cat named Mr. Hemingway.

Other Works by Kirk S Jockell

The Nigel Logan Action Series
See all Titles in the Series Here

The Tales from Stool 17 Series
Finding Port St. Joe (Book 1)
Trouble in Tate's Hell (Book 2)
Dark Days of Judgment (Book 3)

More Nigel Logan Books
Tough Enough (Prequel)
Tupelo Honey (Book 4)
Traffic (Book 5)
Tidewater Moon (Book 6)
Tormented (Book 7)
Trapped (Book 8)

The Cuban (Novella)

Standalone Books

Michael

Made in United States
Troutdale, OR
07/22/2025

33102200R00132